EMOTIONAL HEALING WITH ESSENTIAL OILS

D1366718

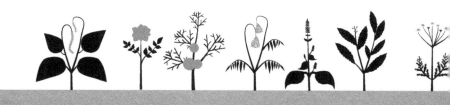

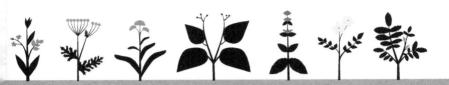

Emotional Healing WITH Essential Oils

RELIEVE ANXIETY, STRESS,
DEPRESSION, AND MOOD
IMBALANCES NATURALLY

Leslie Moldenauer

ROCKRIDGE
PRESS

Copyright © 2019 by Rockridge Press, Emeryville, California

No part of this publication may be reproduced, stored in a retrieval system or transmitted in any form or by any means, electronic, mechanical, photocopying, recording, scanning or otherwise, except as permitted under Sections 107 or 108 of the 1976 United States Copyright Act, without the prior written permission of the Publisher. Requests to the Publisher for permission should be addressed to the Permissions Department, Rockridge Press, 6005 Shellmound Street, Suite 175, Emeryville, CA 94608.

Limit of Liability/Disclaimer of Warranty: The Publisher and the author make no representations or warranties with respect to the accuracy or completeness of the contents of this work and specifically disclaim all warranties, including without limitation warranties of fitness for a particular purpose. No warranty may be created or extended by sales or promotional materials. The advice and strategies contained herein may not be suitable for every situation. This work is sold with the understanding that the Publisher is not engaged in rendering medical, legal or other professional advice or services. If professional assistance is required, the services of a competent professional person should be sought. Neither the Publisher nor the author shall be liable for damages arising herefrom. The fact that an individual, organization or website is referred to in this work as a citation and/or potential source of further information does not mean that the author or the Publisher endorses the information the individual, organization or website may provide or recommendations they/it may make. Further, readers should be aware that Internet websites listed in this work may have changed or disappeared between when this work was written and when it is read.

For general information on our other products and services or to obtain technical support, please contact our Customer Care Department within the U.S. at (866) 744-2665, or outside the U.S. at (510) 253-0500.

Rockridge Press publishes its books in a variety of electronic and print formats. Some content that appears in print may not be available in electronic books, and vice versa.

TRADEMARKS: Rockridge Press and the Rockridge Press logo are trademarks or registered trademarks of Callisto Media Inc. and/or its affiliates, in the United States and other countries, and may not be used without written permission. All other trademarks are the property of their respective owners. Rockridge Press is not associated with any product or vendor mentioned in this book.

Interior and Cover Designer: Emma Hall
Art Producer: Sue Bischofberger
Editor: Vanessa Ta
Production Manager: Riley Hoffman
Production Editor: Melissa Edeburn

ISBN: Print 978-1-64152-546-6 | eBook 978-1-64152-547-3

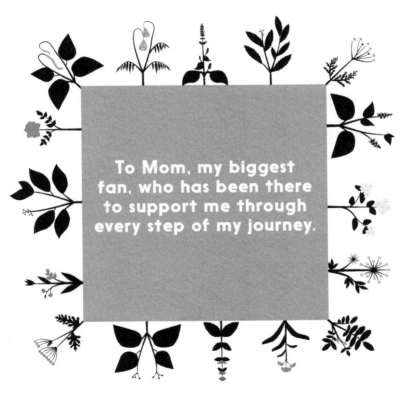

To Mom, my biggest fan, who has been there to support me through every step of my journey.

Contents

Introduction

I stumbled on essential oils more than a decade ago as I worked through the pain of profound loss—first, a little life that I would never get the chance to love and nurture, and then my father a few years later.

I immersed myself in educational courses about complementary and alternative medicine, and I began to realize that oils are so much more than lovely aromas: They are catalysts for recovery. Now, as a lifelong student and devoted aromatherapist, I seek ways to grow from my past and help others, including you, heal.

Emotional healing is not a linear process, and we must be compassionate with ourselves as we learn and mature. As children, we shaped our beliefs and expectations on the basis of the reactions of the adults in our lives. As adults, we filter perceptions of our life events through these conditioned beliefs and expectations, creating anguish. We often lose sight of the fact that we are the architects not only of our adversity but also of our liberation. We have that power.

Increasingly, individuals are looking for natural healing methods offered by essential oils and aromatherapy. Essential oils, in various forms, have been used for centuries. They have been extracted for herbal preparations, resins, gums, ointments, and salves to treat emotional and physical ailments.[1]

Most essential oil enthusiasts know that oils can boost our immune system, speed our recovery when viruses take hold, and even clean our home. But few people know that oils can help heal our emotional psyche. When used appropriately and responsibly, essential oils are a potent adjuvant to our wellness routine.

This book aims to guide you on your path to healing. Be open to the potential of essential oils to increase your resilience to life's stressors by helping you learn that life is happening *for* you, not *to* you. Creating a solid foundation for wellness means focusing on self-care and self-love, and essential oils are critical ingredients to support you along the way.

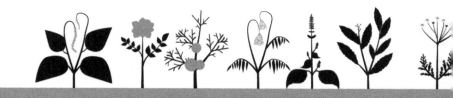

PART 1

Emotional Healing

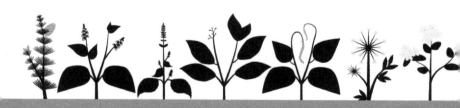

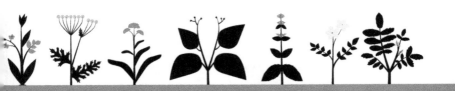

Life can sometimes be tough, handing us grief, loss, change, and upheaval, creating an incredible amount of stress. Essential oils have been found to be an important means of improving mental health.[2] Many studies show their effectiveness. Combined with consistent self-care, essential oils can enrich our lives and improve the state of our overall well-being.[3]

In the coming chapters, I'll discuss the breadth of our emotional landscape and how we can better get in touch with our feelings. I'll also discuss my top 50 essential oils to support your emotional wellness. Last, I provide 100 applications and remedies using those oils. Each remedy is tied to a specific emotional need as well as a desired outcome.

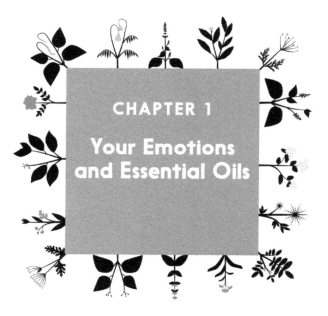

CHAPTER 1

Your Emotions and Essential Oils

Suppressing or ignoring emotions is never healthy. Understanding them and learning how to work through them are essential steps in our personal growth. These steps increase our capacity to heal.

This chapter describes ways to identify and acknowledge your emotions and healthy ways to express them. It will help you understand the essential oil applications that are best suited for you. This knowledge will help you find peace with yourself—and your life.

Knowing How You're Feeling

Many things can disrupt our ability to handle adversity well, including the death a loved one, financial instability, job loss, divorce, a move to a new home, and illness or injury. Even changes that we believe are positive or desired can be viewed as stressful and can affect our health negatively. Difficult events can cause emotional and physiological trauma for years. The earlier we address that trauma, the sooner we can begin to heal and thrive again.

We can begin to understand our feelings by writing in a journal, asking for help, quieting the mind, and being mindful.

WRITING IN A JOURNAL

Journaling is often incredibly therapeutic. Putting pencil to paper and allowing thoughts to flow can frequently help us release strong emotions and give them less power over us. It also can help us find a solution or a way to reframe a situation.

ASKING FOR HELP

Cultivating a strong emotional support network also can make it easier to cope with challenging life events and situations. Speaking with a friend or family member is a great place to start. Keep in mind that although they may have your best interest in mind, they might not be able to help you work through your feelings in the most appropriate or effective ways, especially if you are dealing with serious issues, such as depression. Do not be afraid to seek a qualified professional for help. Many organizations operate free hotlines, offering anonymous services to those in need.

QUIETING YOUR MIND

I do my best thinking when I am able to quiet my mind. When I can calm my thoughts, I am more in tune with my emotions. Then I can begin to see things more clearly.

I am particularly fond of meditation, which I began after my father passed away. Many people, including me, find it difficult to entirely silence their mind. Trust me when I say that even lifelong

Complementary Practices

We know that self-care is crucial to our physical, emotional, and spiritual well-being. At the elementary level, proper nutrition, hydration, and plenty of rest are my top three must-haves every day. Without this foundation—much like a seed in the dirt that does not get food, water, and sun—not much will thrive, including you.

Exercise is essential for not only our overall physical health; for our spiritual and emotional health, moving our body is vital to keep our energy flowing and clear. A few options for movement therapy are walking meditation, yoga, qigong, and slow, intentional rhythmic dance. Doing these exercises with intention and mindfulness is a meaningful and effective path to self-discovery.

Using herbal medicine as a complementary modality is also very beneficial. Unlike essential oils, which do not contain nutrients, herbs are nutrient dense and can support the health of our physical body as well as our spirit. The herb chamomile, for instance, promotes calm, much like the essential oil, but with a plethora of nutrients that also can support our digestive system. Having a cup of tea or using fresh-cut herbs in your meals has a definite benefit.

Acupressure and acupuncture are prized ancient Chinese therapies. According to Chinese medicine, more than 365 points on the human body connect through pathways called meridians. What we consider energy, Chinese medicine considers *qi* or *chi*. Upset or disease in the body results in an imbalance of energy or *qi*, and both acupressure and acupuncture restore its balance and flow. Approaches such as Aroma Acupoint Therapy, developed by aromatherapist Peter Holmes in the early 1990s, combine pure essential oils and acupoints for enhanced treatment.[*]

Reflexology is similar because it focuses on points of the body, particularly on the feet, hands, and ears, but those points correspond to organs of the body rather than energy meridians.

One of my favorite complementary techniques for children and adults alike is Emotional Freedom Technique (EFT), or tapping.[†] Tapping is self-applied on the meridian points while talking through a traumatic memory or stressor to diminish its power.

[*] Snow Lotus, "About Aroma Acupoint Therapy TM," accessed June 5, 2019, www.snowlotus.org/about-aroma-acupoint-therapy-tm/.

[†] The Tapping Solution Foundation, "Promoting the Healing Effects of EFT Tapping to People of All Ages around the World," accessed June 5, 2019, https://www.tappingsolutionfoundation.org/.

yogis experience thoughts when they meditate. But eventually, through practice, I have become more successful at meditation.

Begin by sitting in a comfortable position with your eyes closed. Place your focus on the steadiness of your breath as you inhale and exhale evenly, slowly, and quietly, without pause. Acknowledge any thoughts that enter your mind, and release them instead of addressing them. Try this exercise for just a couple of minutes a day to start. You can lengthen it as you feel able.

Some people enjoy guided imagery and meditation recordings as they relax. Getting outside is another great way to clear your head and quiet your mind. Take a walk and observe nature and wildlife. You might find that you can awaken a deeper understanding of your emotions.

BEING MINDFUL

Mindfulness is a very effective method to train the mind to stay present and calm, according to renowned Zen master Thich Nhat Hanh.[4] His book *Peace Is Every Step: The Path of Mindfulness in Everyday Life* changed my life when I read it more than a decade ago. I returned to it recently when I found myself falling into old patterns of overthinking.

Mindfulness involves training your mind and body to stay in the present moment through breath and practice. It's different from seated meditation and will enable you to cultivate happiness and foster a sense of gratitude, mental states in which we can begin to understand and communicate emotions.

The following Feelings Chart provides a visual for understanding emotions and how they relate to one another. I encourage you to refer back to this chart and use it as a reference tool when you reach part 3 of this book.

Emotional and Physical Health

The connection between physical health and mental health is significant. The World Health Organization defines health as "a state of complete physical, mental and social well-being and not merely the absence of disease or infirmity."* Attaining that state requires focusing on all aspects of our life, including the physical, mental, social, and spiritual aspects. If any of these aspects are neglected, others are sure to suffer.

Poor mental health can and does affect our ability to make the best choices for our overall physical health. It also increases the likelihood of a weakened immune system, opening the door to illness and disease.[†]

Each of us needs to devote time to self-care. Soften the Heart Body Oil (see page 110) will help prepare you to receive this gift. If we stay true to ourselves and honor what we feel in our hearts, shining our light into the world will become easier.

Essential oils and aromatherapy relax the mind, lift the spirit, and remind us to be gentle with ourselves. Nature's wisdom helps us better understand ourselves.

* World Health Organization, "Frequently Asked Questions," accessed June 5, 2019, https://www.who.int/about/who-we-are/frequently-asked-questions.

[†] Ronald Glaser and Janice K. Kiecolt-Glaser, "Stress-Induced Immune Dysfunction: Implications for Health," *Nature Reviews Immunology* 5, no. 3 (2005): 243–51, doi:10.1038/nri1571.

Feelings Chart

ANGRY	AFRAID	NUMB
Frustrated	Anxious	Withdrawn
Embarrassed	Insecure	Unmotivated
Jealous	Dread	Confused
Bitter	Panicked	Detached
Disappointed	Vulnerable	Distant
Resentful	Apprehensive	Empty
Humiliated	Powerless	Uncertain
Annoyed	Terrified	Lost
Livid	Nervous	Overwhelmed
Overwhelmed	Trepidatious	Bored

SAD	EMBARRASSED
Depressed	Ashamed
Hopeless	Guilty
Grief	Rejected
Hurt	Ridiculed
Lonely	Unworthy
Anguish	Humiliated
Empty	Mortified
Melancholy	Discredited
Mournful	Disgraced
Sorrow	Insignificant

Role of Essential Oils

Essential oils are sourced from many parts of a plant (leaves, stems, flowers, bark, and roots), most commonly through steam distillation.

Steam distillation involves passing steam through the plant material, causing the oil sacs to break open and release their contents—a vapor (an oil-and-steam mix). When this vapor cools, the oils separate from the water. Essential oils are the true essence of the plant and are very concentrated extracts, making them powerful, effective, and deserving of our respect. When it comes to essential oils, less is definitely more.

The aroma of essential oils can bring back vivid memories of the past as well as create visceral responses in the body that promote healing. Numerous scientific studies support the effectiveness of essential oils on the limbic system of the brain to lessen stress and assist with anxiety, depression, insomnia, grief, seasonal affective disorder (SAD), post-traumatic stress disorder (PTSD), and much more.[5]

Have you ever wondered why certain smells have the ability to conjure memories and physical feelings so distinctly? These odor and memory links are known as the "Proust phenomenon," in honor of French writer Marcel Proust, who romanticized the memories evoked by the smell of his tea-soaked biscuit in his novel *In Search of Lost Time.*[6]

Research published in 2011 from Utrecht University discovered that when individuals were exposed to an odor and a memory of an important event in their life at the same time, the memory became more vivid.[7] This research shows us that essential oils can and do have an intense, all-encompassing effect on our body and mind. They help bring back old memories so that they can be addressed and create new ones to soothe the spirit. They make us long for their restorative energy time and again and improve the deepening connection with ourselves.

Tools and Containers

If you're not new to essential oils and aromatherapy, you may already have a stocked cabinet with tools and utensils to make my recommended blends. Otherwise, these few things can help get you started.

Diffusers

Having at least one good diffuser is a must in aromatherapy. For safety purposes, I recommend purchasing an ultrasonic diffuser with an automatic shutoff timer to avoid overexposure. Be sure to read package instructions before your first use.

Aromatherapy Inhalers

Aromatherapy inhalers are very inexpensive, discreet, and portable. Put one in your pocket, handbag, backpack, or briefcase to use whenever needed.

Storage Receptacles

Essential oils can degrade with light, air, and warmer temperatures. To avoid degradation, try to purchase bottles that are glass, not plastic, and dark in color such as amber, cobalt blue, or dark green, instead of clear or translucent.

Two- and four-ounce bottles with a simple lid and sprayer top are great to have on hand for your higher-volume creations. Be sure to reuse your jars whenever possible. Clean them with hot water and soap, then run them through your dishwasher on the top shelf, if you have one.

(CONTINUED)

You will want to have both 5 ml dark glass bottles and 10 ml amber or cobalt rollerball bottles on hand for the blends I recommend in the book. If you find something that you love, you can make a larger batch of it to store for later use.

Rollerball bottles are great for on-the-go, quick applications. I prefer stainless steel roller fittings to plastic ones.

Measuring Cups and Bowls

Essential oils will degrade plastic. When purchasing mixing bowls and measuring cups, look for glass or stainless steel. To easily blend larger volumes, make sure you have at least a couple of glass graduated cylinders or beakers to measure in milliliters.

Pipettes

Pipettes are used in scientific laboratories to measure liquids. Inexpensive, one-time-use plastic pipettes are invaluable for your blending space. If you have ever gently tipped your bottle to get a drop or two and had multiple drops come out, then you'll appreciate these handy tools.

*Please also purchase nitrile gloves to avoid exposure to undiluted essential oils.

Your ability to smell comes from 100 million olfactory receptor neurons located in two tiny patches of tissue high up inside your nostrils.[8] These patches of tissue are called olfactory cilia, and they send messages along these neurons to the olfactory bulbs of the brain and then directly to the limbic system. The limbic system also is known as our emotional center and includes parts of our brain that are tied to memory, focus, fear, anxiety, pain, pleasure, and more.[9] With essential oil odor signals going right to the limbic system, it's easy to see how inhaling essential oils affects our emotions.

When we begin to use oils after blending them artfully for their desired chemical constituents, we quickly start to see how they can turn around melancholy, soothe fears, center us, uplift our mood, and promote an overall sense of calm. Simply put, essential oils encourage and support our well-being.

Essential oils have an elemental, natural ability to support the body to do what it has the capacity to do quite well: heal. When we work to address the root cause of our distress in tandem with using essential oils, the benefits are nothing short of miraculous.

Working from a place of prevention is always desirable, but working with a health care professional is best if you have or suspect that you have a more serious mental or physical issue. Be sure to let them know all of the health care measures that you take at home, including essential oils, so that they are properly able to care for you.

The number of individuals prescribed medication for anxiety and depression has reached staggering numbers, so knowing that essential oils can be a very important and effective method of complementary care is more important than ever. Eastern and Western medicine do not need to be exclusive of one another but can be interwoven and work together for the greater good.

Using Essential Oils for Emotional Health

We know that the limbic system of our brain is our emotional center, and essential oils are effective at supporting and promoting emotional wellness. Now, let's look at a few recommended ways to use essential oils.

DIFFUSER

A traditional diffuser is one of the more popular methods used in aromatherapy. Diffusing essential oils in these units is considered passive inhalation and can benefit emotional wellness by reducing stress, uplifting mood, or assisting in a restful night's sleep.

Many types, shapes, and sizes are available for purchase; my preference is a diffuser with a timer for safety. Add distilled water and your oil or oil blend per the manufacturer's instructions. The number of drops will depend on the size of your space. Due to the strength of essential oils and the speed at which they work, diffusing for short times is preferred over diffusing for hours. According to essential oil researcher Robert Tisserand, 30 to 60 minutes of diffusion is ideal for a healthy adult.[10] I recommend shorter times of 10 to 15 minutes for children. Take a break after the timer shuts off the unit before turning it on again to avoid overexposure. Clean the unit well between uses to avoid diffusing old, oxidized oil.

AROMATHERAPY INHALER

Aromatherapy inhalers are available in plastic or a combination of glass and metal, and they have many benefits over a diffuser. Aromatherapy inhalers are user specific, whereas a diffuser exposes everyone in the immediate area to the aroma. Inhalers are discreet and portable so you can take them with you wherever you go. If you get overwhelmed in public spaces, portable inhalers will be of great value to you.

To use, add the essential oils to the cotton wick inside the unit. The aromatherapy inhaler will last three months or more. Cap tightly when not in use.

DIFFUSER JEWELRY

Aromatherapy jewelry is gaining popularity as a method of passive diffusion. Pendant necklaces, as well as bracelets with lava beads, are available in many unique styles and sizes. Apply essential oil to your jewelry on a paper towel, and let it soak in before putting the jewelry on to avoid dropping undiluted essential oil on your skin.

AROMATHERAPY MASSAGE

Do not discount the benefits of aromatherapy massage for emotional wellness. "Massage therapy can improve a person's emotional health by reducing stress and stress [hormones,] by increasing serotonin and thereby reducing depression and pain," according to Tiffany Field, PhD, director of the Touch Research Institute at the University of Miami's Miller School of Medicine.[11] When a massage therapist uses essential oils diluted in massage oil, the client also inhales the aroma, so the essential oil is doing double duty to relax and restore the body, mind, and spirit.

AROMATHERAPY BATHS

Aromatherapy baths are perhaps one of my favorite ways to wind down at the end of a busy day. For your safety, it's important to blend your essential oil in a small amount of carrier oil or a small amount of fragrance-free shampoo or bubble bath before adding it to your bathwater. Not following proper safety precautions could easily cause skin irritation and burning.

See chapter 6 for recipes using these popular aromatherapy methods.

Carrier Oils

A small selection of high-quality carrier oils is important to round out your blending space. Carrier oils are vegetable oils pressed from the fruits, nuts, and seeds of a plant, and they are needed to dilute essential oils before applying them topically to our skin; in fact, the name *carrier oil* was derived from their ability to "carry" oils into the skin.* Vegetable-based carrier oils also are very nourishing to our skin.

Like herbs, carrier oils are nutrient rich and beneficial to our emotional wellness. When making purchases, look for cold-pressed varieties when possible.

My top three recommendations are the following:

Grapeseed oil (*Vitis vinifera*). Pale green to colorless, grapeseed is one of the more popular choices because it easily absorbs into the skin without clogging pores. This oil is nearly odorless, so it will not overpower your senses or your blends. It is an excellent skin care tightener and toner.

Evening primrose oil (*Oenothera biennis*). According to skin care and essential oils expert Susan M. Parker, evening primrose is high enough in gamma linolenic acid to overcome deficiencies and aid hormonal imbalance.[†] This oil is easily absorbed when used in small quantities and blended with other carrier oils. It's the perfect example of a carrier oil being beneficial to both your physical and emotional health.

Jojoba oil (*Simmondsia chinensis*). Technically a wax, jojoba (pronounced *ho-ho-ba*) is an emollient and thus excellent for the skin, providing a light film that holds in moisture yet is nongreasy. Jojoba also protects the acid mantle of our skin, helping guard against skin imbalances.

[*] National Cancer Institute, "NCI Dictionary of Cancer Terms," accessed June 5, 2019, https://www.cancer.gov/publications/dictionaries/cancer-terms/def/carrier-oil.

[†] Susan Parker, *Power of the Seed: Your Guide to Oils for Health and Beauty* (Port Townsend, WA: Process Media, 2015), 138.

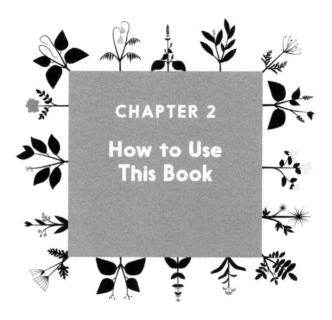

CHAPTER 2

How to Use This Book

This book presents a lot of information, so this section is meant to help guide you about what to expect to get the most out of it. We'll review where we have been as well as what is to come. I'll give an overview of what is covered in later chapters, such as my top 50 essential oils to provide emotional healing, with their safe use as a top priority, and my 100 applications and remedies, with everything from synergies for anxiety (Stop Overthinking Aromatherapy Inhaler, page 101) to remedies for stress (Calming the Nerves Diffuser Blend, page 127) as well as blends formulated specifically for children.

Supporting Your Emotional Wellness

Using this book as it is intended will assist you with incorporating essential oils into your day-to-day routine to support your emotional wellness. A great place to start is to read and begin integrating the many tips from chapter 1. Spend some time going over these concepts and tools to maximize your essential oil use.

Essential oils are meant to be complementary care, and they can be incredibly beneficial for us all. We know how challenging life can be, but we cannot expect essential oils to do all of the work for us. That's why it's important to take a hard look at our current physical and mental states before we begin to move forward.

Journaling, meditation, moving our bodies, and being mindful in everything we do allows us to reach a deep level of understanding so we are better able to communicate to others. A robust social circle is essential in the healing journey. Remember to ask for help when needed. Sometimes a professional can help us work through our feelings.

Being compassionate and kind with ourselves every day as we begin to use essential oil blends will go a long way. Be sure to pay attention to what comes up for you as you start to do the work.

Essential Oil Profiles

In part 2 of the book, you'll find 50 essential oil profiles that can be used for emotional health. For each oil, you'll find the common name and Latin name, a brief description, precautions and safety concerns where applicable, common uses, popular application methods, and healing properties.

Make sure to pay close attention to the precautions. At times, a specific essential oil may need to be avoided if you are taking medication or have a medical condition. A blend also may not be suitable for a child or during pregnancy. Make sure you read all the safety information.

Before you begin creating blends, I also encourage you to study the individual oils to learn as much as you can about them, consider your preferences, and review their emotional health impacts. Remember, essential oils do not affect everyone in the same ways.

Applications and Remedies

In part 3 of the book (page 84), you'll find 100 applications and remedies that are organized by condition or feeling and the desired outcome. Remedies are easily referenced in the General Index (page 209) of the book. You also can search the Conditions Index (page 224) for a particular ailment.

Each remedy will include a descriptive title, preferred method of application, safe age guidelines, and any precautions or contra-indications that apply to an oil or oils in the blend, why the oils were selected, ingredients in the blend, and specific blending instructions where applicable.

Blending is an art form, but as with anything in life, we improve through practice and intention. Your nose will help guide you, so be sure to practice your organoleptic testing as often as you can. A skilled aromatherapist or perfumer can envision how a synergistic blend will smell and what feelings it will evoke before even placing drops in a bottle. They categorize essential oils as having top, middle, or base notes, and blend with these categories in mind. Don't be intimidated. Chapter 5 will cover the principles of essential oil blending with detailed instruction notes. Once you've completed the book, you'll be able to blend the remedies with ease and begin creating unique blends of your own.

You'll likely find that some of the recipes resonate with you more than others, which is to be expected. All of us connect with fragrances in different ways. The key is to find what works best for you.

To help you to make the most out of the book, I have provided two unique and powerful tools: the Emotions Chart and Essential Oils Chart.

The Emotions Chart (see page 197) is an extensive list of emotions relating to emotional wellness benefits you may seek when using essential oils and correlated with specific blends in the book. Use this chart as a tool to find blends that can help get you through the more turbulent moments in life, so you can begin to heal. You can refer to the chart to determine what you need based on your current emotional state and your desired outcome.

The Essential Oils Chart (see page 204) lists the 50 essential oils covered in this book and the negative emotions that they can help address. The chart also lists the desired outcome from using the oil or oil blend. Use this chart to see how your feelings are intertwined and connected and to choose essential oils to support you.

I hope that these tools, among others, and this easy-to-follow guide add to your essential oils knowledge and jump-start your journey to true vitality and wellness.

Testing

Organoleptic testing is a great way to get personal with single oils. The term *organoleptic* refers to using our five senses to analyze oils, but here we are more concerned with the aroma and how it makes us feel.

Be sure your space is quiet and comfortable. Place a drop of oil on a perfume blotter. Close your eyes, and wave the strip about six inches under your nose a few times. What do you think? How does it make you feel? Observe your body. Do not make a judgment; be only a witness. Come back to the blotter a few hours later, and see how you feel then. The aroma may have changed a bit. How about the next day? I invite you to keep a log of your findings. You will be able to identify your favorites in no time.

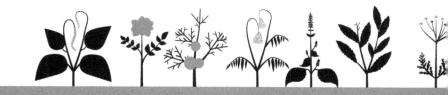

PART 2

Essential Oils for Emotional Work

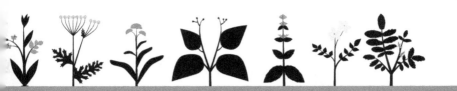

The aromas of essential oils, or their expansive essences, are efficacious for emotional healing. Here are my top 50 preferred oils for working with and through your emotional landscape. Remember, specific essential oils may affect individuals differently, but among the ones in this book, you are sure to find many favorites that will benefit you and your healing. Before we begin exploring each oil's restorative properties, we'll go over safety measures. When you follow basic safety guidelines, you'll greatly reduce any potential risk and greatly increase the effectiveness of your essential oil use.

CHAPTER 3

Using Single Oils

Starting out with essential oils can feel overwhelming, and this chapter will give you general guidelines and essential safety information to get you on your way. What are the pros and cons of using a single essential oil versus a blend of oils? How can we safely apply essential oils to our skin? When diluting essential oils, what are the rules of thumb? You'll find the answers to these questions (and more) along with a dilution chart for easy reference. We'll also cover additional methods for safely using essential oils to avoid risk of injury or adverse effects.

Single Oils versus Blends

Before blending essential oils, it's important to understand them individually so you know their therapeutic benefits and safety risks.

Pinpointing the cause of a reaction is much more difficult once the oils are blended, so knowing their individual traits and how they affect you is important. You can experience a rash from a particular oil when applied topically or discover than an oil is too potent and makes you feel a bit off, although such reactions are rare when an oil is adequately diluted. You may learn that an essential oil intended to be calming instead has an energizing effect on you. You may find that flowery oils are not to your liking but you resonate with tree oils. Even today, nearly 20 years after smelling my first whiff of lavender, I still reach for single oils when immediate emotional support is needed—for instance, when I feel situational anxiety.

For those who are a bit more experienced and have ventured out into the world of published journals and research papers, you undoubtedly have found that the research available to us is typically based on a single oil or an individual constituent of an oil. Analysis rarely discusses a blend of oils, but once you begin blending at home, you'll be addicted to the process and its energetic effects.

Why do we typically blend essential oils rather than use them singly in aromatherapy? To create synergy. In her book *Aromatherapeutic Blending: Essential Oils in Synergy*, Jennifer Peace Rhind explains synergy as "the phenomenon where the effect of the whole is greater than the sum of its component parts."[12]

That said, you *can* add too many oils to a blend. (Once we reach more than five oils, one might say we are going overboard.)

The number of oils depends on your desired aim. If your goal is to create a therapeutic blend but have a pleasant scent—something you would wear as a perfume, for example—three to five oils are ideal. If therapeutics is the end goal, you can safely mix more than five. A set number doesn't exist, but I like to stay on the low end so that all my blends smell amazing. A single essential oil contains 75 different chemical constituents, on average, and I believe that

Safety

With essential oils, nothing is more important to me than safety. I advocate for natural methods of healing whenever possible, and although essentials oils carry some risks, those risks are substantially decreased when safety guidelines are followed.

It's especially important to be aware of oils, such as bergamot, that are photosensitive or phototoxic even when blended with other oils. Although uncommon when blended appropriately, certain essential oils used topically can cause skin damage when exposed to the sun and UV light, including tanning beds. Symptoms can range from blisters to sunburn.

Pregnancy

Essential oils should be used with caution because research shows that small amounts of constituents of essential oils reach the placenta.* If you are considered high risk during pregnancy, avoid essential oil use in the first trimester. You can introduce essential oils during the second and third trimesters, and use them only on an as-needed basis, such as for morning sickness and stress reduction. Shorten diffusing times to 10 to 15 minutes along the lines of my recommendation for young children. Always dilute, and never take essential oils orally during pregnancy.

Babies

As a general precaution, experts agree that essential oil use should be avoided in babies less than three to four months of age, primarily due to their skin permeability.[†] The same safeguard applies to elderly people. This rule of thumb does not mean *carte blanche* usage once your baby is four months old, and I recommend caution during the first year of your baby's life. Introduce oils one at a time.[‡] Please be sure to follow my dilution recommendations. Do not give oils orally to a child.

Immunocompromised

If your immune system is compromised, please use discretion in regard to essential oil use. I recommend a conversation with your health care provider if you would like to use aromatherapy as a complementary treatment.

* Jackie Tillett, and Diane Ames, "The Uses of Aromatherapy in Women's Health," *Journal of Perinatal and Neonatal Nursing* 24, no. 3 (2010): 238–45, doi:10.1097/jpn.0b013e3181ece75d.

† Alice Leung, Swathi Balaji, and Sundeep G. Keswani, "Biology and Function of Fetal and Pediatric Skin," *Facial Plastic Surgery Clinics of North America* 21, no. 1 (2013): 1–6, doi:10.1016/j.fsc.2012.10.001.

‡ Christina Anthis, "Safe Essential Oil Use with Babies and Children," The Hippy Homemaker, August 14, 2014, https://www.thehippyhomemaker.com/essential-oil-safety-babies-children/.

using smaller amounts of individual oils in synergy is more successful for the therapeutic objective.

Lastly, remember your intention behind the blend you are about to make. Clear your space and your mind while blending, so you bottle all of your positive energy, as well. Blend with love and reverence, showing respect to the aromatics that will help you today and in the days ahead.

Neat versus Diluted

The topic of using essential oils "neat," or undiluted on the skin, always seems to be in the spotlight, with camps on both sides. One of the very first things that an aromatherapy student will learn about safety is the importance of diluting essential oils in a vegetable-based carrier oil, for multiple reasons. An advanced practitioner may choose to use oil neat in the case of an emergency but will not teach this method to a beginning student or essential oil enthusiast due to the inherent risk.

The first reason to dilute essential oils before applying them to our skin is for our safety. Every single essential oil available on the market has the potential to cause an adverse reaction on our skin when used undiluted. Even the gentlest, skin-nourishing essential oils can have this effect. For example, although lavender is less irritating to the skin than some other essential oils, irritation can still occur.

Skin irritation is a result of direct contact and is localized to where you applied the oil. The chance of skin irritation is reduced when we dilute oils appropriately, but is still present. Most people will experience a relatively mild reaction, such as reddening of the skin, itching, or burning, whereas others could have more severe reactions, like blistering or painful chemical burns.

A more serious reaction called "sensitization" is more systemic in its etiology and comparable to an allergic reaction to a beesting or specific food.[13] Sensitization can start as a localized reaction where the oil or oil blend was applied, then quickly spread to other areas of the body. Red, blotchy skin; hives; and possible throat swelling can progress, as you would see with any serious allergic reaction. Seek immediate medical attention if you have any of these reactions, and bring the oil(s) you applied to the medical facility. Sensitization is considered a rarity, but the risk increases if essential oils are misused.

When we abuse essential oils by using them improperly or in excess, the potential risk of adverse effect increases. In contrast, when we use essential oils with safety in mind, the risk decreases. I cannot overemphasize taking precautions and using essential oils safely.

The second reason to dilute essential oils in a vegetable-based carrier oil for topical use is because they are volatile organic compounds. The definition of *volatile* in the Merriam-Webster dictionary is "readily vaporizable at a relatively low temperature."[14] What it means for our purposes is that neat essential oils that quickly evaporate will not last on the skin long enough to obtain the desired effect. Vegetable-based carrier oils basically hold down the essential oil, slowing evaporation and allowing for prolonged absorption—similar to the way a delayed-release medication is coated with a substance that prevents the drug from dissolving right away.

Lastly, the sustainability of the plants from which the essential oils are derived is another reason for diluting essential oils. An extremely large volume of plant material is needed to make just one bottle of essential oil, and applying neat or undiluted essential oil results in higher usage. The demand for essential oils continues to rise dramatically, with Global Market Research estimating that the essential oils market will exceed $13 billion by 2024—an astronomical growth projection.[15] We must consider the future of our ecosystem and the essential oils we love if we want to be able to continue to have access to them. If we can reduce usage and lessen the impact by diluting essential oils, then we should.

Every remedy found within this book will be diluted appropriately, similar to the guidelines referenced in the following chart and in accordance with the recommendations made by Robert Tisserand and Rodney Young in their book *Essential Oil Safety*.[16]

AGE RANGE	RECOMMENDED DILUTION OF ESSENTIAL OILS
2 to 12 years	1 percent 5ml (1 drop essential oil to 1 teaspoon carrier oil) 10ml (2 drops essential oil to 2 teaspoons carrier oil)
12+ years	2 percent 5ml (2 drops essential oil to 1 teaspoon carrier oil) 10ml (4 drops essential oil to 2 teaspoons carrier oil)
Temporary, acute health issue	5 to 10 percent 5ml (5 to 10 drops essential oil to 1 teaspoon carrier oil) 10ml (10 to 20 drops essential oil to 2 teaspoons carrier oil)

Note: Please keep in mind that these guidelines are a starting point. They are not strict rules. Adjustments can be made in many instances.

Other Methods

In chapter 1, we covered my top methods for using essential oils, including diffusers, aromatherapy inhalers, diffuser jewelry, aromatherapy massages, and aromatherapy baths.

You might like to try these other fun ways of using your oils:

ANOINTING OIL/PERSONAL PERFUME

I do like to wear perfume, but I am not a fan of synthetic fragrances found on the market. Walking through the fragrance section of a store provides me with an instant headache. I'm not alone; synthetic fragrance sensitivity is common and can result in nausea, headaches, and respiratory issues.[17]

My alternatives are anointing oil and personal perfume.

As far back as biblical times, anointing was a ritual where oils were poured over the head as an act of hospitality and as a form of medicine.[18] Today, anointing is the pouring of aromatic oil over a person's head or massaging oil into the body as a form of self-care. Such is the case in Ayurvedic traditions, where anointing is called *abhyanga,* and the goal is self-love.[19]

Bright and Blissful Anointing Oil (see page 105) is incredibly grounding and healing, with a long-lasting aroma.

Making your own personalized scent also is a lot of fun. Perfumes will last much longer on the skin than the average topical applications because they are formulated with perfumers alcohol versus a carrier oil. Fragrance oils are typically used in perfumery, but you can use the essential oils listed in the book. Try Blissed Personal Perfume (see page 125), guaranteed to turn heads.

ROOM SPRAY

A fine mist of essential oils in a room can help clear energy and provide a respite from the busy world. For home use, a room spray does not need a commercial preservative. Make sure you are using distilled water because tap water spoils faster. You'll also want to use high-proof alcohol in your mixture to adequately dissolve the oil in your base of water. I prefer perfumers alcohol, which you can easily find online. Alternately, you can purchase alcohol like Everclear, if it is available in your state.

A properly formulated spray called Monster Away Room Spray (see page 132) was created to ensure a night of restorative sleep for children with fears at bedtime.

SHOWER MELTS

Shower melts are easy to make, and they store well until ready for use. You'll need baking soda, citric acid, arrowroot powder, distilled water, and essential oils. Form your molds using a fun silicone mold or stainless steel bath bomb mold.

If you have a child who struggles to get up in the morning, make sure to try Oh, Happy Day Shower Melt (see page 103) with them for guaranteed smiles.

STEAM TENT

A steam inhalation of essential oils is very useful during convalescence but also to simply open up the airways and help wake you up. Heat water to below boiling, remove from heat, and pour into a large bowl or a plugged sink. Add three drops of essential oil for an adult or one drop for a child. Cover your head with a towel, close your eyes, and lean over the bowl to inhale the therapeutic steam for several minutes.

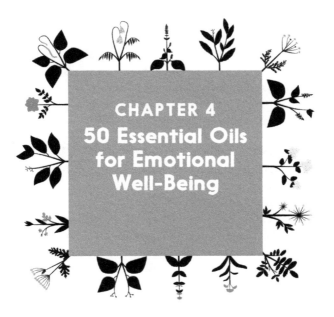

CHAPTER 4
50 Essential Oils for Emotional Well-Being

In this chapter, you will learn all about the 50 essential oils that I have chosen to support emotional well-being. Each oil includes its emotional uses, precautions, general uses, most common applications, and healing medicinal properties—what makes it do what it does.

Angelica Root *Angelica glauca*

Angelica root is steam distilled from the roots of the plant. Energetically, angelica root is a remedy for various traumas, such as PTSD. This emotionally uplifting oil helps release negative, chronic overthinking and worry. Angelica root is useful when overstressed to address anxiety and fear as well as depression.[20]

PRECAUTIONS: According to the International Fragrance Association (IFRA), angelica root is considered a photo-toxic oil, and the maximum dilution ration should remain under 0.8 percent of your total volume.[21] I recommend avoiding sun exposure for 12 to 24 hours if applying this essential oil to your skin.

USES: Angelica root addresses digestive woes by helping stomach upset and increasing appetite when under stress or dealing with situational anxiety. Reach for angelica root when you are feeling unusual amounts of stress or are overanalyzing your current situation.

APPLICATIONS: With a strong, earthy, musky aroma, angelica root is needed in only a small percentage of your overall blend. Due to its strong phototoxic properties, inhalation via diffusion or an essential oil aromatherapy inhaler is the best method of use for this oil. Angelica root is indicated if you are dealing with a past trauma.

PROPERTIES: antianxiety, anti-infective, antispasmodic, carminative, central nervous system tonic, decongestant, diuretic, emmenagogue, expectorant, immunostimulant, stomachic

Balsam Copaiba *Copaifera officinalis*

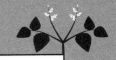

Balsam copaiba is grown deep in the rain forests of Brazil and has a radiant, earthy, and resinous aroma. Copaiba is very beneficial for both anxiety and depression due to its high levels of β-caryophyllene. If you are having troubles with restorative sleep, diffusing copaiba before you lie down at night helps calm the nervous system. Balsam copaiba also is very effective at helping the user handle an underlying trauma.

PRECAUTIONS: This essential oil has no known safety considerations.

USES: ß-caryophyllene is not only effective on an energetic level but also helpful with pain relief. Often it is just as effective, if not more so, for my pain than over-the-counter pain remedies. Lastly, this resin oil provides great support for the respiratory system.

APPLICATIONS: Balsam copaiba is beneficial when applied topically in carrier oil, as a salve for aches and pains, or inhaled for its emotional benefits. If you are emotionally exhausted and tend to have more pain during high-stress moments, a few drops of copaiba essential oil in the bathtub is quite heavenly; try Soothing Bath Salts (see page 135). This oil is a go-to when you need to tap into your intuition, and with a smooth sweet aroma, it is a breeze to blend.

PROPERTIES: analgesic, antibacterial, antifungal, anti-inflammatory, antiseptic, decongestant, expectorant, immunostimulant, nervine, wound-healing

Basil, Sweet *Ocimum basilicum*

Sweet basil essential oil is steam distilled from the leaves of the plant. The essential oil is sweet, herbaceous, and energizing. If you are dealing with mental fatigue and are looking for a boost in endurance to get through the day or a meeting and need to be energetic, confident, and motivated, look for sweet basil to deliver.

PRECAUTIONS: When properly diluted, sweet basil carries no precautions for the user.

USES: Sweet basil is highly antispasmodic and can be applied for various types of pain. If you are suffering from chronic fatigue or adrenal insufficiency, basil should be included in your wellness routine. This oil is a must-have in your blends to help with focus and mental clarity for yourself and your children. Basil is very balanced in its chemistry so it is not overly stimulating but is balancing and expanding.

APPLICATIONS: We can benefit from sweet basil to energize our body and mind in several ways. You can place it in an aromatherapy inhaler, a diffuser, a room spray, a steam tent, a shower melt, or even a refreshing sugar body scrub. Basil is also effective for painful menstrual cramping or digestive upset when it is diluted and rubbed into the abdomen with another antispasmodic, like sweet marjoram. Lastly, if you suffer from chronic knotted shoulders and headaches due to stress, sweet basil will be very beneficial for you.

PROPERTIES: antidepressant, antispasmodic, carminative, energizing, expectorant, immunosupportive, immunostimulant, stomachic

Bergamot Orange *Citrus bergamia*

Bergamot orange is cold pressed from rinds of this citrus fruit and is what some consider an adaptogen, providing the user what is needed for them. This heavenly citrus is one of the most prized essential oils for its ability to provide an uplifting outlook during periods of depression and to reduce emotional and mental fatigue.[22]

PRECAUTIONS: According to the IFRA, bergamot orange is a highly phototoxic essential oil. The IFRA states that leave-on products need to remain under 0.4 percent of the overall volume in your product.[23] I recommend caution with sun exposure for 18 to 24 hours after applying this essential oil to your skin.

USES: The fruity, sweet aroma of bergamot orange is due to the linalyl acetate, which reduces inflammation and irritation, helping address minor aches and pains.[24] Bergamot orange essential oil is a carminative, useful for indigestion, flatulence, and colic.[25] Put it to good use during times of situational anxiety and depression, including SAD.

APPLICATIONS: The most effective method of use for this essential oil for emotional wellness is via inhalation for emotional and mental fatigue. Even though bergamot orange is highly phototoxic, it has clear benefits to the skin when blended with caution. Bergamot orange is listed in Breast Health Synergy (see page 182). Several studies also support the use of citrus oils high in limonene as an anti-cancer agent.[26]

PROPERTIES: antianxiety, antibacterial, antidepressant, anti-infective, anti-inflammatory, antispasmodic, antiviral, carminative, central nervous system tonic, digestive stimulant, sedative, stomachic

Bergamot Mint *Mentha citrata*

Bergamot mint essential oil is steam distilled from the leaves of the plant. This oil is a perfect light and fresh blend of minty citrus and is sure to be a hit with everyone in your home. Bergamot mint can be used on its own to address tension, stress, and anxiety, and it works wonders to perk up low mood.[27] When looking to find balance and clarity, reach for bergamot mint.

PRECAUTIONS: When blended appropriately, bergamot mint is generally a safe essential oil. Unlike bergamot orange, the mint variety of bergamot is not considered a phototoxic essential oil.

USES: Bergamot mint is useful in blends to reduce muscle spasms and calm minor aches and pains. Bergamot mint also is a must-have for children to boost low mood or to help their anger fizzle out. It is one of the only mints that are not energizing, so it can help you unwind after a long day. The chemistry of bergamot mint is similar to a combination of lavender and bergamot, so it is a beautifully balanced essential oil, providing the user with harmony and stability.

APPLICATIONS: Bergamot mint is a great choice in an aroma bath or bath ball for all ages but especially for young children. It is beneficial with all methods of inhalation, whether in a diffuser, an inhaler, or a steam tent. Use this essential oil topically to reduce tension, stress, and anxiety.

PROPERTIES: analgesic, antidepressant, anti-infective, anti-inflammatory, antiseptic, antispasmodic, carminative, central nervous system tonic, deodorant, immunosupportive

Black Pepper *Piper nigrum*

Black pepper, with the tangy aroma of freshly ground pepper-corns, has numerous emotional benefits, including increasing concentration, encouraging grounding to Mother Earth, and providing solace to those who need to work through fears and inspire change.[28] Black pepper also has mild aphrodisiac properties, helping couples connect and rediscover intimacy.

PRECAUTIONS: Black pepper is warming when applied to the skin; therefore, it has the potential to irritate those with sensitive skin. I would not recommend this oil in a bath, where increased absorption is likely on more sensitive areas.

USES: This warm and peppery essential oil stimulates circulation and can soothe nerve, joint, or muscular pain.[29] If pain increases due to stress, having this essential oil on hand is a good idea. Black pepper also supports a healthy digestive system.[30] If you get an upset stomach from situational anxiety, black pepper can be part of your belly oil.

APPLICATIONS: Inhale black pepper to remain alert and focused. This oil can be over-powering for some on its own, but once blended with other essential oils, it is quite lovely. This oil, which is sourced primarily in Madagascar, contains both ß-caryophyllene and ß-pinene, which help reduce pain and calm inflammation.[31] Apply topically, properly diluted, to areas of need. Some experts use this oil in a blend to support smoking cessation and subsequent periods of withdrawal.[32]

PROPERTIES: anti-inflammatory, antiseptic, antiviral, carminative, digestive stimulant, expectorant, febrifuge, rubefacient, stimulant

Black Spruce *Picea mariana*

Black spruce essential oil is steam distilled from the needles of the *Picea mariana* evergreen tree. The invigoratingly sweet and crisp aroma of black spruce is dynamic in its emotional uses and superb for the mental exhaustion that comes with stress-related endocrine challenges. According to Kurt Schnaubelt, author of *Medical Aromatherapy: Healing with Essential Oils,* "the polycyclic terpenoid compounds have a tonic effect on adrenal, thyroid, and pituitary glands, providing hormonal equilibrium."[33] Tree oils bring us a greater connection to the earth, the roots, and ourselves.

PRECAUTIONS: Black spruce essential oil is generally very safe. It does, however, have a strong aroma, so only a drop or two is needed when using in a diffuser or an aromatherapy inhaler.

USES: Black spruce is beneficial when you are chronically stressed and emotionally exhausted. If you suffer from adrenal fatigue, hypothyroidism, or chronic fatigue syndrome, this essential oil will be very healing for you. Black spruce is revitalizing and expanding but also gentle in the way that it restores energy and strengthens resolve. It will not be overly stimulating.

APPLICATIONS: This tree oil can support our physical body in a muscle rub for common aches and pains. Black spruce is a welcome addition to most essential oil applications, including various inhalation methods and applied topically if properly diluted. You also can try a couple of drops in an aroma bath when your nerves are feeling a bit frazzled.

PROPERTIES: analgesic, antianxiety, antibacterial, antifungal, anti-inflammatory, antioxidant, antispasmodic, diuretic, mucolytic, warming

Blue Tansy *Tanacetum annum*

Blue tansy is steam distilled from wildflower tops grown in the Moroccan countryside. Also called Moroccan chamomile for its fresh, rich, slightly herbaceous scent, this essential oil reminds me of standing in an apple field. Blue tansy is a rich color of blue due to its aromatic chemical constituent chamazulene. This essential oil is noted for reducing worry and overthinking. Blue tansy encourages patience and knowing when to slow down, tune in, and listen to our inner wisdom.[34]

PRECAUTIONS: This essential oil has no known safety considerations. Use this oil sparingly in your blends for sustainability purposes. Purchase only what you intend to use.

USES: Blue tansy essential oil is useful for emotional upset, such as frustration, agitation, and irritability. When you find your patience is running thin, or realize you are worrying and overthinking more than usual, take advantage of blue tansy's ability to quiet your mind and help you regain your focus.

APPLICATIONS: Blue tansy can be used in a diffuser at home or an aromatherapy inhaler on the go. Only a couple of drops are needed in an overall blend. Blue tansy also can be put to work in an aroma bath to treat situational anxiety. Try blue tansy with lavender essential oil to prepare you for a restorative night's sleep.

PROPERTIES: analgesic, anti-allergic, antianxiety, anti-asthma, antihistamine, anti-inflammatory, calming, nervine, sedative, wound-healing

Buddha Wood *Eremophila mitchellii*

Buddha wood essential oil, which is distilled from a shrub native to Australia, is an earthy, woody, and resinous essential oil that is deeply grounding and encourages introspection. This oil is perfect during moments when you feel ungrounded and detached. If you are working on being more mindful throughout the day, be sure to use this essential oil. Buddha wood also can be used as an adequate replacement for Indian sandalwood, which has sustainability concerns.

PRECAUTIONS: This essential oil has no known safety considerations.

USES: Buddha wood essential oil is sure to provide you with the ultimate Zen feeling. This essential oil also is helpful to reduce the common aches and pains of daily life that are magnified in our body when we are under stress.[35] Place a small amount in a massage oil to promote inner peace and relaxed muscles.

APPLICATIONS: Whether diffused or placed in an aromatherapy inhaler, the aroma of Buddha wood will sweep away your troubles. Its woodsy scent provides respite during meditation or yoga and is quite effectual to cleanse the energy in any space. Buddha wood is heavenly when applied to the skin, and its high viscosity increases the aroma's staying power. Try Release the Anger Aromatherapy Inhaler (see page 109) to soothe your heart and ground your body and spirit.

PROPERTIES: analgesic, antianxiety, antidepressant, anti-inflammatory, calming, immunosupportive, sedative

Cardamom *Elettaria cardamomum*

Cardamom essential oil is steam distilled from the seeds of the plant. Traditionally known as the queen of the spices, cardamom has a scent that is spicy and enticing.[36] Cardamom is incredibly soothing and nurturing during times of sadness and depression, including those gray, gloomy days of winter. This oil is also beneficial for the worrier-type personality in finding stillness from mind chatter.[37]

PRECAUTION: According to *Essential Oil Safety*, oils high in 1,8-cineole should be kept away from the face of any child under the age of 10.[38]

USES: Cardamom essential oil supports a healthy digestive system. If your stomach is the first to react to anxiety, this oil can provide relief.[39] Cardamom is very warming in nature. Apply it to the skin properly diluted to bring warmth to the area, increasing circulation to reduce aches and pains. This oil's warmth also benefits the respiratory system, opening the airways. Feel open, refreshed, and clearheaded with cardamom essential oil.

APPLICATIONS: Warming and stimulating, this oil may be used in an inhaler or a belly rub to support digestive woes, especially nausea. Cardamom essential oil is beneficial for many application methods, including in a bath, inhaled in an aromatherapy inhaler or diffuser, and applied directly on the skin when properly diluted. Look for cardamom used with rose otto in my Finding Respite Bath Blend (see page 179) for the ultimate self-care experience.

PROPERTIES: antiemetic, anti-infective, antispasmodic, carminative, digestive stimulant, digestive tonic, diuretic, expectorant, stomachic, warming

Cedarwood Atlas *Cedrus atlantica*

Standing under a canopy of cedar trees, taking in the amazing aroma, and feeling the power of their presence is truly a breathtaking experience. Cedar trees can grow over 100 feet tall and live more than 1,000 years; seemingly nothing can topple these unwavering giants.[40] Cedarwood atlas essential oil can provide this feeling for you, too: grounding, endurance, strength, and resilience. Know how powerful you are with this stunning essential oil.

PRECAUTIONS: This essential oil has no known safety considerations. Cedarwood atlas is an oil that has significant sustainability concerns. I recommend buying only what you will use, and use it sparingly.

USES: Cedarwood atlas is indicated when you are feeling insecure, vulnerable, and disconnected from your true self. This captivating tree oil is standing by to help strengthen your resolve and light the way back to your authenticity. Use this tree oil to support clearer breathing and mental expansiveness. This is one of my number one go-to oils for children. You can begin using this essential oil at six months of age.

APPLICATIONS: Cedarwood atlas can be used in practically all areas and with all methods of application. The most effective method is inhalation; an aromatherapy inhaler would be my preference unless illness is present, in which case a steam tent may be more effective. Cedarwood atlas is a powerful fixative in skin care blends.

PROPERTIES: antibacterial, anti-infective, astringent, carminative, diuretic, expectorant, sedative, wound-healing

Chamomile, Cape *Eriocephalus punctulatus*

This lovely essential oil is steam distilled from the buds and flowers of the cape chamomile plant. I love using this species of chamomile when I am feeling overwhelmed with a to-do list the size of Texas, and it encourages me to be mindful when I am worrying about the future. The lovely fruity aroma of this oil is perhaps the most relaxing of all essential oils.

PRECAUTIONS: This essential oil has no known safety considerations.

USES: Cape chamomile can help bring you back to homeostasis when feeling irritable, jittery, or angry. Parents often burn the candle at both ends, leaving themselves feeling frazzled and unbalanced and wondering how to manage everything. Cape chamomile is high in esters, a fragrant organic compound, so it is profoundly therapeutic, encouraging serenity and peacefulness. Wind down at the end of your day with this soft and cool floral aroma in your diffuser and a cup of tea to ensure a beautiful night of sleep.

APPLICATIONS: Include cape chamomile properly diluted in your skin care products to keep you feeling centered throughout the day. Add it to an aroma bath to forget all of your troubles before bedtime. Try Clear and Composed Fizzy Bath Ball (see page 97) during dips in your monthly cycle to provide you a much-needed break. Lastly, use cape chamomile in a diffuser or aromatherapy inhaler to help you stay in the present moment.

PROPERTIES: antianxiety, anti-inflammatory, antispasmodic, cooling, sedative, wound-healing

Chamomile, Roman *Chamaelmelum nobile*

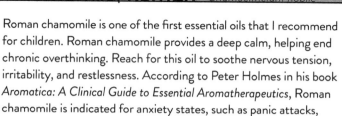

Roman chamomile is one of the first essential oils that I recommend for children. Roman chamomile provides a deep calm, helping end chronic overthinking. Reach for this oil to soothe nervous tension, irritability, and restlessness. According to Peter Holmes in his book *Aromatica: A Clinical Guide to Essential Aromatherapeutics*, Roman chamomile is indicated for anxiety states, such as panic attacks, various phobias, bipolar disorder, and PTSD.[41]

PRECAUTIONS: This essential oil has no known safety considerations.

USES: Put Roman chamomile to use when you anticipate a situation that is anxiety provoking. One of the more common symptoms of stress is stomach upset. Roman chamomile has strong antispasmodic properties and is a digestive tonic, so use it with any ailment of the digestive system, including bloating, colic, gas, and indigestion. Roman chamomile is composed of primarily esters, which are calming sedatives that are useful to combat muscle spasms, relieve PMS symptoms, and release stress and tension resulting in headaches and knotted shoulders.[42]

APPLICATIONS: Roman chamomile is included in Muscle Calm Massage Oil (see page 134) to release tension in the body. In addition to massage, try Roman chamomile and lavender in your child's bath before bed to assure a soothing and restorative night's sleep. Lastly, keep an aromatherapy inhaler in your bag, briefcase, or backpack to promote relaxation and stability.

PROPERTIES: analgesic, antianxiety, anti-asthma, antidepressant, antispasmodic, central nervous system tonic, digestive tonic, sedative, stomachic

Cistus   *Cistus ladaniferus*

Cistus, also known as rock rose or labdanum, has a warm, rich, and spicy aroma and is a must-have in a diffuser when performing yoga, meditation, or other forms of energy work. It also has been used after traumatic events to protect the heart and nourish and settle the adrenal glands.[43] The popular flower essence Rescue Remedy from Bach Remedies contains primarily rock rose for this purpose.[44]

PRECAUTIONS: This essential oil has no known safety considerations.

USES: Cistus essential oil is beneficial for addressing old emotional wounds of the heart in addition to current ones. I recommend using this oil, if possible, during counseling or therapy. Cistus has a unique chemical profile, including various monoterpenes that support its use as a nervous system tonic and have analgesic and anti-inflammatory properties.[45]

APPLICATIONS: Use cistus with other skin-nourishing oils, such as helichrysum, myrrh, or lavender, to soothe the skin and quiet the mind. Cistus essential oil is an important oil in a diffuser or inhaler for any type of energy work to encourage opening and softening of the heart and mind. It also is helpful after shock or trauma.

PROPERTIES: analgesic, antibacterial, anti-infective, anti-inflammatory, antimicrobial, antioxidant, antiseptic, antiviral, astringent, expectorant, mucolytic, nervine, sedative, tonic, wound-healing

Clary Sage *Salvia sclarea*

Clary sage has a woodsy, floral, fruity, and slightly herbaceous aroma and is primarily grown and distilled in France. Clary sage is beneficial for our emotions, especially when we feel out of balance. Look for clary sage to help bring into balance feelings of irritability, weepiness, and even melancholy connected to hormonal fluctuations.[46]

PRECAUTIONS: This oil should be used with caution while pregnant. Clary sage can promote a strong relaxation response, so please make sure you know how it affects you before having an alcoholic beverage or getting behind the wheel.

USES: Clary sage relieves the emotional aspects of the menstrual cycle as well as the physical ones. PMS symptoms, including cramps and headaches, and menopausal symptoms, such as hot flashes and insomnia, all benefit from a little clary sage. If you struggle with insomnia, make sure to include clary sage with other sedative oils for a night of good sleep.

APPLICATIONS: Take an aroma bath with clary sage when you feel out of sorts. Only a couple of drops help bring the body back into homeostasis. You may benefit from blending a body oil with clary sage and lavender the entire week before your expected estrogen dip to reduce symptoms before they start.

PROPERTIES: antianxiety, antidepressant, anti-inflammatory, antispasmodic, astringent, carminative, central nervous system tonic, digestive tonic, hormone balancing, nervine, sedative, stomachic, tonic, uterine tonic

Cypress *Cupressus sempervirens*

Cypress is a conifer tree oil with a fresh and herbaceous aroma. All conifer essential oils have an affinity to the endocrine system and help bring balance and stabilization to the thyroid gland and adrenal glands.[47] The properties that we can draw from these tree oils strengthen our resolve, helping us heal.

PRECAUTIONS: This essential oil has no known safety considerations.

USES: Cypress essential oil, above all other conifer oils, has a very strong affinity to emotional healing, specifically in terms of sadness, grief, and loss. Cypress also helps you ease anxiety and embrace new paths in life, such as a career change or new home. Put this essential oil into action during any transition in life.

APPLICATIONS: Cypress oil can do double duty for your emotional well-being when you apply the diluted oil topically over your adrenal glands and inhale it at the same time. Try Clear Expression Aromatherapy Inhaler (see page 176) to draw strength to support your nervous system. You also can take advantage of the amazing aroma of cypress as part of your housecleaning routine. The combination of cypress and lemon essential oils is a great disinfectant for your home, and it smells good, too.

PROPERTIES: antibacterial, antiseptic, antispasmodic, astringent, decongestant, diuretic, central nervous system tonic

Davana *Artemisia pallens*

Davana may not be a familiar essential oil, but you will love it once you know more about its benefits and have the opportunity to use it. Davana often smells quite different in the bottle than on the skin, and it will likely smell different on your skin than on someone else's, which is likely due to pheromone differences. Look to davana to lift low moods and put a smile on your face again.[48]

PRECAUTIONS: This essential oil has no known safety considerations.

USES: Davana essential oil is used in perfumeries due to its sensual, rich, and fruity aroma. This essential oil has an affinity to the female reproductive system. Similar to clary sage, davana can assist in balancing hormones and managing both PMS and menopausal symptoms.[49] The difference in this regard is that davana is very uplifting whereas clary sage is sedating.

APPLICATIONS: Davana can be worn on your wrists diluted on its own or blended with other essential oils for a beautiful personal perfume. Ready to give it a try? Blend Blissed Personal Perfume (see page 125), and try it for yourself. Place a couple drops of davana in a diffuser during moments of unrest in your monthly cycle, or add it to a bath blend to help improve low mood and increase optimism.

PROPERTIES: antianxiety, antidepressant, antiseptic, antiviral, emmenagogue, expectorant, wound-healing

Elemi *Canarium luzonicum*

Elemi is a lemony, spicy, and warm essential oil steam distilled from the tropical flowering elemi tree in the Philippines rain forest. This essential oil is energetically uplifting and clarifying. The word *elemi* in Arabic means "as above, so below" and can be loosely translated to "on earth, as it is in heaven" or "we are all one, namaste."[50] The general meaning is oneness, an understanding of our true nature, and a respect and reverence for one another and ourselves.

PRECAUTIONS: This essential oil has no known safety considerations.

USES: Be sure to include this resin oil in your skin care routine for bright and youthful skin.[51] It promotes an overall serene feeling without being a strong sedative. Elemi is a strong fixative, with therapeutics useful for ceremonial purposes. This oil is a superior choice if working to move stuck energy, to have a breakthrough from a trauma or loss, or if you are feeling withdrawn. Elemi can help you find acceptance and peace.

APPLICATIONS: Elemi is a useful addition to a skin toner or in a compress to help calm and soothe irritated skin. Use elemi essential oil in a diffuser, an aromatherapy inhaler, or even in a luxurious bath to clear the mind and to be open to the mysteries of the universe and that over which we have no control. Try Good Spirits Aromatherapy Inhaler (see page 118).

PROPERTIES: analgesic, antibacterial, antifungal, anti-inflammatory, antiviral, expectorant, sedative, tonic

Fragonia *Agonis fragrans*

Fragonia is the only essential oil to date that is trademarked. The plant is grown in the Australian bush, and the oil is distilled from the leaves and twigs of the flowery shrub. Fragonia is a very balanced essential oil in its chemical constituents, and it helps bring life into balance, as well.[52] Look to Fragonia to work not only in the present moment but also with events of the past. It can help you reset old patterns and leave behind things that no longer serve you.

PRECAUTIONS: This essential oil has no known safety considerations.

USES: Fragonia essential oil on an energetic level helps bring about balance and harmony to your emotional being. This oil is incredibly safe for kids; use it to boost the immune system and support cases of cold, cough, and other flu-type symptoms.[53] Fragonia is similar in its chemistry to tea tree, with a much softer, pleasing scent to soothe tired, stressed-out muscles.

APPLICATIONS: Make sure to have Fragonia on hand if you have small children. Add it diluted to the bath to help kids wind down after a busy day. It is not only useful in a diffuser to stop the spread of illness but also extremely supportive of restful sleep. Try Dreamy Night Diffuser Blend (see page 157) in your favorite diffuser tonight.

PROPERTIES: analgesic, anti-asthma, antifungal, anti-inflammatory, antimicrobial, antiviral, decongestant, expectorant, immunostimulant

Frankincense *Boswellia sacra*

Frankincense sacra resin is carefully harvested from trees in Oman. The oil has a bright, warm, resinous, and earthy aroma, superb for meditation and other energy-based practices. Frankincense is protective, purifying, and grounding; use it to cleanse the energy in your space or when you need introspection and courage to heal old traumas.

PRECAUTIONS: This essential oil has no known safety considerations.

USES: Longtime British aromatherapist Shirley Price suggests frankincense to address generalized symptoms of stress, including muscular tension and spasms, headaches, aches and pains, and digestive stress, and to keep the immune system robust and strong.[54] This variety of frankincense also lends itself to instances of situational anxiety and depression. Frankincense is supportive of aging skin; add a couple drops to your existing face serum or moisturizer.

APPLICATIONS: Frankincense is great for all skin types when properly diluted. Diffuse in the home to help stop the spread of virus and bacteria. Lastly, when doing any kind of restorative energy work or counseling, use frankincense via inhalation to keep you protected and grounded and ready to confront anything.[55] Before your next yoga, meditation, or journaling session, make up a bottle of Clear the Energy Room Spray (see page 116) to set the stage for clearing out stagnant energy and self-limiting thought patterns.

PROPERTIES: analgesic, antianxiety, antidepressant, anti-inflammatory, antimicrobial, antispasmodic, immunosupportive, expectorant, sedative, tonic

Galbanum *Ferula galbaniflua*

Galbanum essential oil is steam distilled from the resin of the flowering plant *Ferula galbaniflua* and has a very strong green, weedy, and slightly sweet aroma. Some think it is reminiscent of green bell peppers. Due to its intense aroma, use it sparingly to avoid overpowering your blends. Jennifer Peace Rhind notes in her book *Aromatherapeutic Blending: Essential Oils in Synergy* that galbanum combined with black spruce or pine essential oil is beneficial for adrenal insufficiency and overall support of the nervous system.[56]

PRECAUTIONS: This essential oil has no known safety considerations.

USES: Galbanum is favorable for our skin, particularly for revitalizing aging skin when it is used with elemi in skin products.[57] In her book *The Encyclopedia of Essential Oils,* aromatherapy expert Julia Lawless says that galbanum can be used for a wide variety of digestive upset, including discomfort caused by anxiety.[58]

APPLICATIONS: A massage with diluted galbanum directly over the adrenal glands while inhaling via a diffuser or an aromatherapy inhaler is useful to aid in rebalancing the nervous system. I recommend using this aromatherapy inhaler in combination with deep breathing to center you during moments of unrest. One drop in an overall blend is likely all that is needed for stomach upset. If you are ready for a nervous system boost, try Rejuvenation Diffuser Blend (see page 131).

PROPERTIES: anti-asthma, anti-inflammatory, anti-microbial, antiseptic, calming, carminative, emmenagogue, expectorant, sedative, wound-healing

Geranium *Pelargonium graveolens*

Geranium essential oil, with its floral, sweet, and heady aroma, is very versatile with many benefits. When you are feeling melancholy or just need a pick-me-up, you will find geranium to be incredibly balancing, uplifting, and revitalizing.

In *Aromatherapy for Healing the Spirit: Restoring Emotional and Mental Balance with Essential Oils*, U.K.-based aromatherapist Gabriel Mojay says geranium can help with imbalances that manifest as stress, restlessness, or fear. He says, "A combination of geranium and orange oils is called [for] to pacify the will and ease frustration."[59]

PRECAUTIONS: This essential oil has no known safety considerations.

USES: Geranium essential oil has an affinity to the skin. You can add the oil to your existing skin or hair care routine to deeply nourish areas of concern, such as the scalp, face, neck, and chest.[60] When diluted in a carrier oil, geranium essential oil can assist with minor aches and pains.

APPLICATIONS: Geranium is a wonderful addition to your existing skin care routine for glowing, healthy skin. Include geranium essential oil in aromatherapy inhalers and diffusers as well as add it to an aroma bath with clary sage or davana during dips in your monthly cycle. Try Restore Tranquility Aromatherapy Inhaler (see page 130) next time you feel out of sorts.

PROPERTIES: antianxiety, antibacterial, antidepressant, antifungal, anti-inflammatory, antimicrobial, antispasmodic, hormone balancing, sedative, tonic

Grapefruit *Citrus paradisi*

Grapefruit essential oil has a bright and fresh fruity aroma that is sure to please even the pickiest of noses. Reach for this gem when you need help getting out of a rut. This oil is great for moments of low energy, sadness, or depression, or for when you are just plain grumpy.[61] Grapefruit essential oil will provide the sparkle to help bring back your cheerful self once again.

PRECAUTIONS: Grapefruit essential oil is phototoxic. According to the IFRA, the maximum dilution for wash-off products is 4 percent.[62] If you apply grapefruit essential oil topically at a level higher than the recommended 4 percent, avoid sun exposure for 12 to 24 hours.

USES: Like cistus, which also contains linalool, grapefruit can assist in boosting the immune system and help regulate the normal flow of the lymphatic system. Researchers from the Niigata University School of Medicine in Japan found that inhaling the scent of grapefruit can activate sympathetic nerve activity and help control appetite.[63] This is great news!

APPLICATIONS: Diffuse grapefruit essential oil in a room to help remove the presence of any unwanted microbial activity and halt the spread of illness. Or, to brighten your mood, try Bright and Cheerful Diffuser Blend (see page 115) with a dynamic combination of citrus oils. If you would like to try grapefruit to combat food cravings, try Stop the Cravings Aromatherapy Inhaler (see page 139).

PROPERTIES: antianxiety, antibacterial, antidepressant, anti-inflammatory, antioxidant, astringent, immunostimulant, lymphatic decongestant, tonic

Helichrysum *Helichrysum italicum*

Helichrysum is a must-have for every home that uses essential oils as a complementary modality. Having gone through grief, loss, and adrenal exhaustion, I can say that helichrysum was critical to my wellness. It addresses situational anxiety and depression, lethargy, and nervous system exhaustion, and it helps encourage homeostasis in the body and mind.[64]

In her book *Subtle Aromatherapy*, Patricia Davis writes, "Helichrysum induces feelings of compassion, and is called for to activate the intuitive side of our brain when meditating or performing guided imagery."[65]

PRECAUTIONS: This essential oil has no known safety considerations.

USES: Use diluted helichrysum on the third eye when performing any kind of energy work. Reach for *italicum* over other varieties for its affinity to the integumentary system. Helichrysum also is indicated for individuals who have experienced trauma, especially when forgiveness is needed.

APPLICATIONS: If you are dealing with situational anxiety or depression, apply diluted helichrysum to the skin or use it in an aromatherapy diffuser or inhaler to help console you. Helichrysum can be added to your favorite bath blend to address nervous exhaustion and lift your mood. Be sure to try Gain Perspective Aromatherapy Inhaler (see page 168) to assist your healing.

PROPERTIES: analgesic, antidepressant, anti-inflammatory, antiseptic, antispasmodic, tonic, wound-healing

Hemp   *Cannabis sativa*

Hemp essential oil is not to be confused with marijuana. Only terpenes—no cannabinoids or THC—cross over in the distillation process. Hemp oil's aroma is very herbaceous and earthy, much like the plant itself.

According to the *Handbook of Cannabis Therapeutics from Bench to Bedside*, the compounds in cannabis do not need to be absorbed systemically through the lungs to provide calming and sedative effects.[66] Hemp oil, which offers a softening of your body and mind, is very useful for situational stress and anxiety.

PRECAUTIONS: This essential oil has no known safety considerations.

USES: Hemp essential oil contains constituents with analgesic and anti-inflammatory properties, making it helpful topically for aches and pains as well as skin conditions, such as contact dermatitis, eczema, and psoriasis.[67]

APPLICATIONS: Hemp essential oil can be found in many personal care products on the supermarket shelves because of its affinity to the skin. If you have any trouble areas, try applying hemp diluted in carrier oil with

helichrysum to find relief. If stress tends to cause more aches and pains than usual, try Muscle Calm Massage Oil (see page 134) to calm and soothe any overly irritated areas. You also can use a variety of inhalation methods, including aromatherapy inhalers and diffusers.

PROPERTIES: analgesic, antibacterial, antifungal, anti-inflammatory, antiseptic, decongestant, expectorant, immunostimulant, nerve tonic, wound-healing

Jasmine Absolute *Jasminum grandiflorum*

Jasmine is a base note in aromatherapy and has a heady, exotic, sweet, and intense floral aroma. To some, the aroma is over-powering, but I assure you it is divine when artfully blended. Jasmine is used heavily in perfumery and has aphrodisiac qualities for both the wearer and the recipient. Don't say I didn't warn you.

Jasmine is a well-known antidepressant and sedative. If you have moments in life when you are despondent; feeling sadness, grief, or anger; or feeling perhaps even a bit fragile, look for jasmine to help provide solace, hope, and aid to soften the heart.[68]

PRECAUTIONS: The IFRA recommends a maximum dermal limit of 0.7 percent to avoid possible skin irritation.[69]

USES: In *The Encyclopedia of Essential Oils*, author Julia Lawless writes that jasmine has an affinity to the reproductive system, acting as a uterine tonic and helping menstrual issues as well as sexual diffi-culties.[70] Jasmine is a nervous system sedative, helping calm the parasympathetic system when adrenaline takes over during highly stressful moments.

APPLICATIONS: Jasmine mixes very well with citrus; add these oils to a diffuser or aromatherapy inhaler to uplift the spirit. Add jasmine absolute with a fixative, like vetiver or Australian sandalwood, and any citrus oil to the bath. My favorites are sweet orange or red mandarin. Be sure to try Pampered and Peaceful Bath Ball (see page 180).

PROPERTIES: antianxiety, antidepressant, antispasmodic, aphrodisiac, calming, sedative, strengthening

Ho Wood *Cinnamomum camphora var. linalool*

A few essential oils are derived from various parts of the cinnamomum camphora tree found in Asia. Ho wood is different from ho leaf, ravintsara, and other varieties of camphor that all come from this same tree.[71] It also carries the highest amount of linalool of any steam-distilled essential oil.

Linalool is widely known to have sedative properties, and I like to think of ho wood as a provider of peace and tranquility. Look to use ho wood with general stress and anxiety if you have reached the point of burnout, as it is a potent nervous system tonic. Ho wood is a masterful essential oil to include in your next yoga class, meditation, or any other energetic practice you participate in.

PRECAUTIONS: This essential oil has no known safety considerations.

USES: Ho wood can be used with other sedating essential oils to help during moments of anger or panic, and it can serve as a part of your child's bedtime routine. Upon inhalation, you'll feel your mind slow, your breath steady, and your heart rate lower quite quickly.

APPLICATIONS: Whether you apply topically, inhale, or place in a warm bath, the fresh and woody scent of ho wood is sure to bring serenity. Try Snug as a Bug in a Rug Diffuser Blend (see page 159).

PROPERTIES: analgesic, antianxiety, antibacterial, antifungal, anti-inflammatory, antispasmodic, calming, sedative

Laurel Leaf *Laurus nobilis*

Laurel leaf is steam distilled from the leaves of the shrub, which grows primarily in Bulgaria and Turkey. The oil is similar to clove in its scent, but it's a gentler, smoother aroma that has fresh, strong, spicy, and sweet tones all rolled into one. From an emotional standpoint, laurel leaf is unique. It is a warming and uplifting feel-good oil, helping anyone who suffers from negativity and low self-esteem.

PRECAUTIONS: According to experts Robert Tisserand and Rodney Young, the maximum dilution ratio when applying to the skin is 0.5 percent.[72]

USES: You can use laurel leaf essential oil for a wide range of immunosupportive actions to assist cold and flu recovery, among other viral infections. Add it to a blend to support the respiratory system. Julia Lawless also suggests that this essential oil might be beneficial for loss of appetite.[73]

APPLICATIONS: Laurel leaf could be used in a diffuser, steam tent, or warming bath when illness has taken hold to both recover faster and stop the spread of germs. Alternatively, inhale a blend with this essential oil when you are feeling low, lack confidence, or want to harness laurel leaf's positive energy. This slightly spicy essential oil is a welcome addition to focus blends if you're feeling all over the place. Try Rejuvenation Diffuser Blend (see page 131) to help provide a pick-me-up when you are in need.

PROPERTIES: analgesic, antibacterial, anti-inflammatory, antimicrobial, antioxidant, antispasmodic, antiviral, carminative, digestive tonic, immunosupportive, tonic

Lavandin *Lavandula × intermedia 'Grosso'*

Lavandin, primarily grown in France, imparts an aroma somewhat similar to lavender but with sharper camphoraceous notes. Lavandin typically is used for soap and other uplifting personal care products. It does not produce the extreme sedative calm of its cousin lavender.[74] Lavandin has antidepressant and anxiolytic properties, providing a sense of ease and mental strength not gained from many oils.

PRECAUTIONS: When properly diluted, this essential oil has no known safety considerations.

USES: Lavandin is a tonic for the nervous system, helping address frayed nerves much like a vitamin B complex. Try using lavandin via inhalation as well as topically for nervousness and other, more serious nerve conditions. The goal here is to provide support. This essential oil also has analgesic properties, helping reduce pain and inflammation. It may help address headaches produced by stress and tension.

APPLICATIONS: When applying diluted lavandin to the skin, concern is minimum. If you like to make soap or lotion at home, try lavandin in place of lavender. Lavandin is an excellent addition to a pain blend or skin tonic. Add lavandin to a bath to soothe your nerves and your worries. Inhalation also is a very effective method of using lavandin. If you find yourself feeling very frazzled, try Calming the Nerves Diffuser Blend (see page 127) in your favorite diffuser.

PROPERTIES: analgesic, antianxiety, antibacterial, antidepressant, antifungal, anti-inflammatory, antimicrobial, antioxidant, antiviral, calming, immunostimulant, sedative

Lavender *Lavandula angustifolia*

Lavender is grown in gardens all over the globe for its intoxicating, sweet aroma and a multitude of uses. By far, lavender is one of the most popular essential oils today due to its aroma and versatility. Lavender essential oil is a sedative and is indicated during times of stress and situational anxiety.[75] Overall, the oil is balancing and softening, providing the user with a sense of ease, assurance, and contentment.

PRECAUTIONS: This essential oil has no known safety considerations. Please make sure you purchase yours from one of the trusted sources included in the Resources section of this book (page 195). Because of its high demand, suppliers often adulterate it.

USES: Lavender essential oil is beneficial to the skin; it is nourishing, purifying, and healing. If you are dealing with any type of pain, be sure to include lavender in your pain blend to apply topically. Lavender is one of the most common essential oils recommended for stress.

APPLICATIONS: Lavender essential oil is a perfectly suitable stand-alone. Wave the bottle directly under your nose or place a drop on your child's favorite blanket or teddy bear for quick results. Apply it topically, in a bath, or in your dresser or closet to freshen your clothes. Give Release the Pressure Aromatherapy Inhaler (see page 128) a try during your more tense moments.

PROPERTIES: analgesic, anti-anxiety, antibacterial, antidepressant, antifungal, anti-inflammatory, antimicrobial, antispasmodic, antiviral, calming, immunostimulant, sedative, wound-healing

Lemon *Citrus limon*

Lemon essential oil is sweet, fresh, and incredibly vibrant. Choose this essential oil to help nudge you out of low energy, moments of sadness or anxiety, and situational depression. Look to lemon essential oil to energize, revitalize, and bring good thoughts back to mind.

PRECAUTIONS: According to the IFRA, cold-pressed lemon essential oil is phototoxic. The IFRA states that leave-on products need to remain less than 2 percent of the overall volume in your product.[76] If you apply lemon essential oil topically at a higher level than the recommended 2 percent, be sure to avoid sun exposure for 12 to 24 hours. Lemon essential oil in a glass of water often is recommended for ingestion, but this combination is unsafe.[77] Do not use it that way.

USES: Lemon essential oil is effective for SAD and is being used in health care settings to reduce worry and fear associated with that clinical diagnosis.[78] Lemon is your answer if you are looking to boost the immune system for everyone in the home, lift mood, and purify your space.

APPLICATIONS: Inhalation is the most recommended use in a diffuser, in an inhaler, or right out of the bottle in a pinch. Lemon essential oil is ideal in household hard-surface cleaners. If you are looking to use lemon essential oil topically, purchase the steam-distilled variety to avoid worrying about the phototoxic component.

PROPERTIES: antianxiety, antibacterial, antidepressant, antifungal, antioxidant, antiseptic, antispasmodic, antiviral, astringent, carminative, immunostimulant, lymph decongestant, tonic

Lime *Citrus aurantifolia*

Emotionally speaking, lime essential oil is bright, vibrant, and uplifting. Add lime essential oil to your favorite diffuser to help children focus while doing homework or wake up and prepare for the day ahead. Reach for lime essential oil for stress as well as situational anxiety and depression. Inhaling this oil during the gloomy days of winter also has been shown to help lift the spirits.

PRECAUTIONS: According to the IFRA, lime essential oil (cold pressed) is phototoxic, and more than 0.7 percent in a blend should not be applied to the skin in a leave-on product.[79] If you apply this essential oil topically at a level higher than the recommended 0.7 percent, avoid sun exposure for 12 to 24 hours.

USES: Much like the other citrus oils, lime essential oil is very revitalizing. Some people have great results using lime for minor indigestion and stomach upset. Diffuse it in the home to stop the spread of unwanted germs.

APPLICATIONS: The steam-distilled variety of lime is not phototoxic and is quite heavenly when applied to the skin in an oil, lotion, or sugar scrub. Add lime essential oil to an aromatherapy inhaler to increase focus and concentration or cut through the congestion that may come with viral illnesses. If you have a child who occasionally struggles with completing homework, try Homework Time Diffuser Blend (see page 148).

PROPERTIES: antianxiety, antibacterial, antidepressant, antioxidant, antiviral, astringent, digestive tonic, immunostimulant, lymph decongestant, tonic

Mandarin, Red *Citrus reticulata var. mandarin*

Of all the varieties of mandarin essential oil, red has by far the sweetest aroma. If you have a child who is very particular about smells, this essential oil is likely to be a winner in their book. Red mandarin is fresh and fruity and supportive of emotional well-being.[80] This essential oil helps remove blocked stagnant energy when you are feeling stuck and unable to move forward. If you are struggling to be kind and compassionate with yourself, inhaling red mandarin will gently coax you to find your center.

PRECAUTIONS: Unlike many of the citrus essential oils, red mandarin does not have a phototoxic component.

USES: Make the most of this tonic for the central nervous system during times of situational anxiety and depression to bring an overall sense of calm and contentment, encouraging self-compassion. Red mandarin essential oil also is beneficial for our physical body and is one of my preferred oils for children. It also may calm the stomach and increase the appetite during periods of emotional upset.

APPLICATIONS: When someone falls ill in the home, place red mandarin in the diffuser to combat germs and help promote clear breathing. Need help finding your center? Place Finding Solace Diffuser Blend (see page 107) in your favorite diffuser.

PROPERTIES: analgesic, antianxiety, antibacterial, antidepressant, anti-inflammatory, antioxidant, antispasmodic, antiviral, carminative, central nervous system tonic, digestive tonic, expectorant, immunostimulant, sedative

Marjoram, Sweet 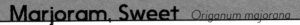 *Origanum majorana*

Sweet marjoram is distilled from the flowers and leaves of the herb. According to Gabriel Mojay in his book *Aromatherapy for Healing the Spirit*, "Marjoram helps calm obsessive thinking, ease emotional craving and promote the capacity of inner self-nurturing."[81] Sweet marjoram is one of the oils I recommend to support you during deeply sorrowful times of grief and loss.

PRECAUTIONS: This essential oil has no known safety considerations.

USES: Sweet marjoram is highly antispasmodic; use it to soothe pesky muscle spasms, menstrual cramping, and growing pains.[82] This warming oil helps revitalize sore, tired muscles. If you are a worrier and tend to overanalyze situations, try inhaling sweet marjoram essential oil; it can strengthen your resolve and calm the unsettled mind at the same time. Sweet marjoram is a great addition to a blend to help calm the kiddos at the end of a busy day.

APPLICATIONS: Make sweet marjoram a staple in your favorite pain blend to find long-lasting relief. Add a few drops to a diffuser, an aromatherapy inhaler, a steam tent, massage oil, or a bath to enjoy this sweet and camphorous essential oil. If you suffer from persistent aches and pains, blend some Stress Ache Body Oil (see page 136) and alleviate your ills. You can add a warm pack to the skin after application to enhance the oil's effects.

PROPERTIES: antibacterial, antifungal, anti-inflammatory, antimicrobial, antioxidant, antispasmodic, antiviral, calming, hypotensive, immunostimulant

Myrrh *Commiphora myrrha*

Myrrh essential oil has a sweet, balsamic, and slightly spicy aroma. If you have an overthinking or type A personality, reach for this oil to remain peaceful, focused, and centered. Myrrh essential oil is incredibly dynamic and is used in spiritual practices, such as realigning the chakras, reiki, and other forms of energy work.[83] Keep myrrh close by if you are feeling numb or stuck and are looking for clarity about a situation.

PRECAUTIONS: According to experts Robert Tisserand and Rodney Young, myrrh essential oil may be fetotoxic due to the presence of ß-elemene and furanodiene; avoid it during pregnancy and while breastfeeding.[84]

USES: Myrrh is a central nervous system tonic; make sure to include it in your daily routine if you are feeling very fatigued or have been diagnosed with endocrine challenges. Myrrh may not be the first oil we consider for the overthinking and overanalyzing mind, but it can be very effective in a blend with vetiver or petitgrain.

APPLICATIONS: Make myrrh a staple in your skin care routine. Adding a couple of drops to an evening face serum to balance and nourish your skin is superb. Apply diluted myrrh to any trouble areas to encourage cell regeneration and healing. Include myrrh in a diffuser or aromatherapy inhaler when stress levels are high and you need help slowing down.

PROPERTIES: analgesic, antibacterial, antifungal, anti-inflammatory, anti-microbial, astringent, calming, expectorant, mucolytic, wound-healing

Neroli *Citrus aurantium var. amara*

Neroli has an exotic and sweet orange, floral scent that imparts sensual, euphoric impressions. This oil is one of aromatherapy's best-kept secrets as the ultimate stress eliminator. Neroli has an affinity to the crown chakra, representing higher knowledge and universal energy.[85] If you are feeling withdrawn, distant, and unsure of yourself and your place in the world, look for neroli to help you discern and discover your purpose.

PRECAUTIONS: This essential oil has no known safety considerations. Neroli is costly due to the volume of blossoms required to obtain even a small amount of oil. As a result, the oil is frequently adulterated; know your supplier.

USES: Neroli is known for being an energetic essential oil that supports emotional wellness, but it is very healing for the physical body, as well, and is used widely in perfumery and skin care products. This blissful oil can help reduce inflammation on this skin, reduce redness and irritation, and soothe burns and minor wounds.[86]

APPLICATIONS: I recommend blending neroli essential oil in small amounts to use on the skin. You will be pleased with the results. If using in a diffuser or an aromatherapy inhaler, a little bit will go a long way. Try Crown Chakra: Higher Source Rollerball Blend (see page 194) to experience the energy of this dynamic essential oil to soothe the spirit and quiet mental chatter.

PROPERTIES: analgesic, antianxiety, antibacterial, antidepressant, anti-inflammatory, antioxidant, antispasmodic, aphrodisiac, immunosupportive, nervine, sedative, tonic

Orange, Sweet *Citrus sinensis*

Sweet orange essential oil is cold pressed from the rinds of this jeweled fruit, and its alluring aroma is a favorite of many essential oil professionals and enthusiasts. Several studies show the effectiveness of this oil as an anxiolytic. One from 2018 showed that inhaling orange prior to dental procedures significantly reduced anxiety.[87] I consider sweet orange a universal essential oil as it blends beautifully with nearly all other oils.

PRECAUTIONS: Unlike many of the citrus essential oils, sweet orange does not have a phototoxic component.

USES: Sweet orange is a potent antianxiety and antidepressant essential oil. Inhale sweet orange as a mood enhancer and relaxant; it is very balancing and harmonizing in nature. If stress has your stomach tied in knots, orange will be an ally to help release the tension.

APPLICATIONS: Whether inhaled from a diffuser or an inhaler or applied topically to the skin, sweet orange essential oil is sure to be a quick favorite. Add a couple drops to a damp towel in the dryer to freshen linens. A blend of oils properly formulated in a spray bottle is sublime to brighten a room and shift the energy in your space. Grab the supplies listed in Clear the Energy Room Spray (see page 116) to create a safe and effective essential oil spray.

PROPERTIES: antianxiety, antibacterial, antidepressant, antiseptic, antispasmodic, antiviral, carminative, digestive tonic, disinfectant, stomachic, tonic

Palo Santo *Bursera graveolens*

Palo santo, also called holy wood, is a smoky, spicy essential oil that has historically been used in spiritual traditions as a part of energy clearing and keeping away evil. Burning the wood from the palo santo tree has been practiced for centuries, much longer than plant distillation as we know it today.[88] Palo santo essential oil is used for energy clearing and protection, meditation, and assisting with focus and concentration.

PRECAUTIONS: According to Robert Tisserand and Rodney Young, the recommend dermal maximum of palo santo is 3.4 percent.[89]

USES: Palo santo can be used topically when properly diluted for aches and pains, particularly, headaches and stress-related migraines, due to its analgesic and anti-inflammatory properties.[90] This oil also is beneficial for supporting a healthy respiratory system, opening the airways, and enhancing breathing. Put palo santo to use at the end of a hectic day to clear the energy.

APPLICATIONS: Palo santo is a must-have in the diffuser or aromatherapy inhaler for promoting focus, concentration, mind clearing, and respiratory health. Apply it topically in a carrier oil for aches and pains, especially headaches. Palo santo would be a dynamic addition to a personal perfume or anointing oil.

PROPERTIES: analgesic, antianxiety, anti-asthma, antibacterial, antidepressant, anti-inflammatory, anti-oxidant, antispasmodic, central nervous system tonic, decongestant, expectorant, immunosupportive, tonic

Patchouli *Pogostemon cablin*

When you think of the sweet, earthy, and peppery aroma of patchouli essential oil, it may remind you of the 1960s and the generation of free love. Hippies loved their patchouli oil, which is notable for its potent pheromone and anti-stress properties.

PRECAUTIONS: This essential oil has no known safety considerations.

USES: Patchouli has a way of arousing good vibes and promoting feelings of blissful contentment without being a strong sedative. It also bolsters the immune system. If you are looking to obtain an overall vibe of true contentment and happiness, make sure you are inhaling patchouli oil.

APPLICATIONS: If you'd like to make a personal perfume scent, patchouli provides a great base. Since the oil is so thick and viscous, applying patchouli to the skin will do double duty when inhaled and will remain on the skin longer than other oils. If you're placing it in a diffuser, be sure to clean the unit thoroughly after use to keep the oil from (literally) sticking around. Try Embracing Femininity Bath Salts (see page 161) for a unique self-care experience.

PROPERTIES: antianxiety, antibacterial, antidepressant, anti-inflammatory, antiseptic, deodorant, sedative, tonic, wound-healing

Petitgrain *Citrus aurantium var. amara or bigaradia*

Petitgrain has a light floral aroma with sweet undertones. This oil is steam distilled from the leaves and twigs of the same tree as neroli blossoms, so the aromas are similar, but petitgrain is less expensive. It's the first oil I reach for when my oldest child has trouble falling asleep because he can't stop his thoughts and feels frustrated.

Longtime aromatherapist Patricia Davis writes that although neroli "evokes the highest psychic or spiritual levels of mind, [petitgrain] relates more to the conscious, intellectual mind. Inhale this oil when you need mental clarity."[91]

PRECAUTIONS: This essential oil has no known safety considerations.

USES: Petitgrain has a variety of uses, including lessening pain and discomfort, soothing an upset stomach, and stopping the spread of germs. It can remove odors from rooms and also is a tonic for the central nervous system.

APPLICATIONS: Petitgrain essential oil in a spray bottle can cleanse the air of microbes, disinfect hard surfaces, promote peace in the home, and support a night's good sleep. Be sure to make Stop Overthinking Aromatherapy Inhaler (see page 101), which is ideal for children and adults. Blend a couple drops of petitgrain with orange and a small amount of patchouli for an unbeatable bath experience.

PROPERTIES: analgesic, antianxiety, antibacterial, antifungal, anti-inflammatory, antimicrobial, antioxidant, antispasmodic, antiviral, immunostimulant, nervine, sedative, tonic

Pink Pepper *Schinus molle*

Pink pepper essential oil is fresh, sweet, peppery, and spicy. Because it's quite different from black pepper, it's sometimes called "false pepper." This little gem is not as well known as some of the other oils, but it helps soothe spirits and calm thoughts while enhancing alertness and expansion.[92] I have used this oil with bergamot and lemon for situational anxiety and depression and had fantastic results.

PRECAUTIONS: This essential oil has no known contraindications. Since this is a warming essential oil, I would caution against using it in a bathtub.

USES: Pink pepper can help increase appetite after a period of convalescence, lessen nausea, and help soothe a stressed and upset stomach. This essential oil is a rubefacient; it creates warmth when applied to the skin, so use it to combat common aches and pains. The chemical constituents of pink pepper can work with your body to soothe and relax the nervous system, which is perfect during times of stress and situational anxiety.

APPLICATIONS: Pink pepper essential oil, whether used topically on the skin or inhaled via a diffuser or an aromatherapy inhaler, is sure to settle the nerves while putting a little pep in your step. It's safe for all ages; try The Sun Will Come Out Diffuser Blend (see page 111) on challenging, gloomy days.

PROPERTIES: anti-inflammatory, antiseptic, antiviral, carminative, digestive, expectorant, rubefacient, stimulant

Rhododendron *Rhododendron anthopogon*

This particular species of rhododendron is different from the common plant that grows in the United States. According to aromatherapist Virginia Musacchio of Stillpoint Aromatics, "Rhododendron is a very powerful essential oil in working with energetic issues related to the fourth chakra, namely those of the heart and lungs. The leaf is where a plant breathes, respires, and takes in its life force. This is a reminder for us to breathe deeply and live fully. Oils that are distilled from the leaf also protect us from negativity and support expansion."[93]

Rhododendron supports our blossoming like a flower, helping us be brave, go for our goals, and manifest our desires. Inhale rhododendron to help birth the next chapter of your life.

PRECAUTIONS: This essential oil has no known contraindications.

USES: A study in rodents showed that rhododendron exhibited adaptogenic properties and increased their resilience under specific stress models.[94] Rhododendron supports the endocrine system, and the oil supports our resilience to stress, as well.

APPLICATIONS: Rhododendron can be used in a diffuser or aromatherapy inhaler. Add this oil to skin care blends to nourish and balance all skin types. If you are looking to rediscover your creative space, try Bright and Blissful Anointing Oil (see page 105).

PROPERTIES: analgesic, antianxiety, antibacterial, antidepressant, antifungal, anti-inflammatory, antioxidant, antispasmodic, decongestant, immunostimulant

Rose Otto *Rosa × damascena*

Rose otto is an exquisite, deep bouquet of rosy sweetness. If I could recommend only one essential oil to use during times of loss and radical grief, it is rose otto. Rose represents love, purity, and passion. The detailed patterns of the rose petals, and the depth and layers of one complex flower, resemble the complexity and uniqueness of our hearts. The delicate rose helps us heal our emotional wounds.

PRECAUTIONS: According to Robert Tisserand and Rodney Young, rose otto has a maximum dermal ratio of 0.6 percent.[95]

USES: Rose otto supports our overall well-being. We often close off our heart as a form of protection when we are hurting, and rose otto helps restore self-esteem and encourage forgiveness of ourselves and others.

APPLICATIONS: Apply rose otto essential oil topically to your skin while being mindful of the maximum dermal recommendation to avoid any potential skin irritation. Inhalation of this heavenly floral is beneficial, using a diffuser, an aromatherapy inhaler, or a steam tent. Place a couple drops of rose and cardamom essential oils in the bathtub or try Soften the Heart Body Oil (see page 110) during periods of grief and loss.

PROPERTIES: antianxiety, antibacterial, antidepressant, anti-inflammatory, anti-microbial, antioxidant, antispasmodic, aphrodisiac, astringent, hormone balancing, nervine, sedative, tonic

Ruh Khus *Vetiveria zizanioides*

Ruh khus essential oil, also known as wild vetiver, is known to benefit those suffering from anger, anxiety, and depression, as well as an inability to concentrate, fatigue, insomnia, and irritability.[96] It's also called nature's tranquilizer and has an intense, earthy, rich, and slightly balsamic aroma. If you like vetiver essential oil, you will love ruh khus.

PRECAUTIONS: This essential oil has no known safety considerations.

USES: This essential oil is popular in perfume shops in India for its rich, earthy scent and its fixative properties. Reach for ruh khus to freshen any area, including a stinky gym bag. Add ruh khus to your blends for situational anxiety and depression to help reduce aggravation and frustration.

APPLICATIONS: Ruh khus blends well with helichrysum or lavender to nourish inflamed or aging skin. From my own clinical experience, it also can help treat blemishes. Place the oil in an aromatherapy inhaler or diffuser to help increase concentration and melt away your frustrations. To calm angry feelings, blend my Release the Anger Aromatherapy Inhaler (see page 109) and breathe it in and out.

PROPERTIES: antianxiety, antidepressant, antirheumatic, deodorant, immunosupportive, nervine, sedative, wound-healing

Sandalwood, Australian *Santalum spicatum*

Australian sandalwood's vanillalike, sweet, resinous, and full-bodied aroma has a strong ability to support our emotional wellness. This variety is quite sustainable, unlike *Santalum album* of India. In fact, western Australia is home to the world's largest sustainable sandalwood plantation, a reported 617,000 square miles, or roughly three times the size of France.[97] Australian sandalwood helps give us the courage to speak our truth with kindness and compassion while upholding healthy boundaries.

PRECAUTIONS: This essential oil has no known safety considerations.

USES: Australian sandalwood has sedative effects and is helpful for stress and situational anxiety and depression. It also helps release nervous tension. Aromatherapist Gabriel Mojay writes that sandalwood's "soft, woody aroma helps reduce incessant overthinking and encourages our realigning with inner peace and unity."[98]

APPLICATIONS: Blend Australian sandalwood in a carrier oil for an aromatic massage oil, encouraging circulation and lymphatic flow and instilling inner calm. Place one drop in a bowl of steamy water and inhale to settle irritated coughs. Soak in a tub with sandalwood and red mandarin for an utterly sublime self-care ritual. Wear alone or blend with other essential oils as a unique personal scent.

PROPERTIES: analgesic, antianxiety, anti-inflammatory, antispasmodic, antiviral, central nervous system sedative, central nervous system tonic, nervine, sedative, wound-healing

Siberian Fir *Abies sibirica*

Siberian fir has a fresh and sweet pine aroma. Trees often are symbols of healing, and tree essential oils are incredibly grounding and help us revitalize and restore our roots.[99] This essential oil helps calm overthinking, ease worry, and return us firmly and steadily to our body.

PRECAUTIONS: This essential oil has no known safety considerations.

USES: Siberian fir has positive energy to bring you strength during times of difficulty and struggle. If you want to be more positive about something that is happening in your life or need to make an important decision surrounding your life's path, Siberian fir can help. Be mindful of the fact that tree oils represent unwavering strength and strong roots. Include this tree oil in your life for increased resilience.

APPLICATIONS: Use this oil alone or with other oils in a diffuser or an aromatherapy inhaler to bring you strength and peace. Steam tents also are indicated with this oil. Siberian fir also helps boost the immune system when under stress, so include it in your favorite diffuser when illness is present. Try Protector Diffuser Blend (see page 166) when someone in the house falls ill.

PROPERTIES: analgesic, anti-inflammatory, antirheumatic, antiseptic, circulatory stimulant, disinfectant, expectorant, mucolytic, rubefacient

Spikenard *Nardostachys jatamansi*

Distilled from the roots of the *Nardostachys jatamansi* plant in Nepal, this earthy, woodsy essential oil can help you find stability in turbulent times. Spikenard essential oil is used in aromatherapy primarily as a tonic for our nervous system and to provide healing for our heart.[100]

PRECAUTIONS: This essential oil has no known safety considerations. However, sustainability is an issue, so purchase from one of my recommended suppliers who harvest the roots ethically so the plant can continue to flourish.

USES: If you are suffering from situational anxiety, you have been hurt, your heart needs your compassion, or you need to attain forgiveness for yourself or others, make this oil a part of your wellness plan. Combine with other essential oils, such as balsam copaiba, clary sage, lavender, or neroli, that have sedative properties. Lastly, if stress and anxiety afflict you, add Spikenard to your pain blends for relief.

APPLICATIONS: Spikenard can be applied topically when diluted, inhaled in a diffuser or an aromatherapy inhaler, or placed in an aromatherapy bath. Look for Blissfully Sleepy Diffuser Blend (see page 154). Diffuse 30 minutes before bedtime.

PROPERTIES: antianxiety, antifungal, anti-inflammatory, antispasmodic, calming, central nervous system tonic, sedative

Vetiver *Vetiveria zizanioides*

Vetiver essential oil is distilled from the roots of the *Vetiveria zizanioides* plant and has a unique deeply rich and earthy aroma. I have found that on its own, vetiver can be overpowering, but when artfully blended, it is quite lovely and very effective. Vetiver is touted as being an essential oil that helps provide focus, and although vetiver slows the hyperactive mind, its magic is in helping us reconnect with ourselves by providing reassurance and self-confidence.

PRECAUTIONS: This essential oil has no known safety considerations.

USES: Reach for vetiver if you lean toward perfectionism under stress. Vetiver helps restore faith in yourself and remind you that mistakes are okay. In his book *Aromatica*, Peter Holmes writes that vetiver supports our immune system, helps balance hormones, and assists with restoring our digestive system.[101]

APPLICATIONS: Use vetiver in any skin care blend as a deodorizer or an antifungal or as a rich addition to a perfume blend. Vetiver is great in a wide range of inhalation methods as well as in an aromatherapy bath to wind down at the end of the day. Vetiver is used with lime and a few other oils to help with focus in Homework Time Diffuser Blend (see page 148).

PROPERTIES: antibacterial, antidepressant, antifungal, anti-inflammatory, deodorant, immune supportive, nervine, sedative, tonic

Yarrow *Achillea millefolium*

The white flowering tops and green leaves of the *Achillea millefolium* plant create a rich, herbaceous-scented essential oil. The chemical constituent chamazulene is what gives the oil its stunning blue color. Emotionally, yarrow helps us handle anger that is connected to a life event or a trauma.

PRECAUTIONS: This essential oil has no known safety considerations.

USES: Yarrow helps us release negative feelings by going through them, not around them.[102] This blue oil reduces inflammation and pain, so you can apply it topically to muscles and joints to alleviate discomfort. Yarrow acts on our digestive system much like other blue oils high in chamazulene, helping with upset stomach, gas, indigestion, and irritable bowel syndrome in times of high stress.

APPLICATIONS: Yarrow works with subtlety, but its effects are undeniable. Apply diluted yarrow essential oil topically in case of spasms or tight muscles to find quick relief. Put yarrow in an aromatherapy inhaler or diffuser to assist with feelings of anger and frustration. Try yarrow with helichrysum and others in Gain Perspective Aromatherapy Inhaler (see page 168).

PROPERTIES: analgesic, anti-inflammatory, antioxidant, antispasmodic, antiviral, carminative, digestive tonic, immunostimulant, sedative

Ylang-Ylang *Cananga odorata*

Ylang-ylang is a super sweet, tropical, fruity, and floral essential oil that is ideal for skin care. Some call ylang-ylang a "poor man's jasmine" because they are both very heady florals with very different price tags. Peter Holmes writes in *Aromatica* that ylang-ylang is used for mood swings, nervous tension, fearfulness, low self-esteem, and loss of libido, among other conditions.[103]

PRECAUTIONS: According to Robert Tisserand and Rodney Young, the maximum dilution ratio when applying ylang-ylang to the skin is 0.8 percent.[104] A little bit will go a long way with this floral oil; excessive inhalation via diffusion can result in headache and nausea.

USES: Look for this essential oil to foster calm, relaxation, and contentment. Its intoxicating aroma promotes sensual awakenings.

APPLICATIONS: Ylang-ylang is recommended for its aphrodisiac properties. Add it to a hot bath or body oil for a romantic and relaxing massage. Some people also say that ylang-ylang, like clary sage, has a mild euphoric effect. Preparing for date night? Whip up Lagging Libido Diffuser Blend (see page 162).

PROPERTIES: analgesic, antianxiety, antidepressant, anti-inflammatory, antiseptic, aphrodisiac, hypotensive, nervine, sedative, tonic

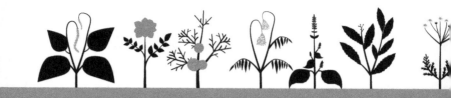

PART 3

Applications for Well-Being

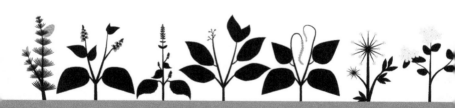

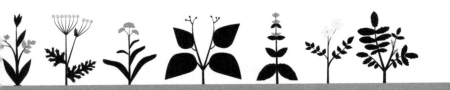

Many of the oils described here hold a special place in my heart because they have helped me learn and grow, and they will support you in your journey as well.

Now the fun part: learning how and when to use essential oils. Before we explore applications and remedies, we will delve into some of the fundamentals of the art of blending these powerful healing catalysts. This information will empower you to begin using your oils with confidence and conviction.

CHAPTER 5

Making Blends

We have so many available options and variations for blending with essential oils, and finding synergy among them is an important key to success. Briefly, synergy is the idea that the therapeutic effect of combined essential oils is more effective than any one oil alone, and that concept is especially significant when you are blending for emotional wellness.

This chapter will discuss when blending is appropriate and the differences between blending and layering your oils. Some additional principles of blending are provided that will be very helpful for you to know in order to use the recipes in this book and to create your own. I'll also review some basic safety guidelines.

When to Blend

Essential oils trigger feelings, old and new, and have a powerful ability to support our emotional wellness. Using essential oils and perfume blotters to create a wonderful-smelling therapeutic blend is a beautiful form of art. Your hands and your olfactory senses will become seasoned with practice, and you'll eventually develop natural instincts for how oil blends will smell before you even put them together.

When you sit with individual oils before beginning to blend with them, it's easier to distinguish how they will affect you and whether you like them or not. You do not need to be an expert at blending essential oils to get started; all you need are the right tools and safety awareness.

Blending for emotional wellness has many benefits. For instance, if you need a blend to calm your mind but also wake you up, you can curate a blend using multiple essential oils. Two examples are Good Spirits Aromatherapy Inhaler (see page 118), which is safe for children ages 5 and up, and Be Hopeful Rollerball Blend (see page 112), formulated just for children.

Another great reason to blend with essential oils is aroma. This way, some of the more potent essential oils can be blended in smaller amounts so you can reap their therapeutic benefits without being overpowered by their aromas.

Other times, I use a single essential oil instead of a blend. For instance, I may reach for a bottle of lavender and breathe in its heady floral aroma when I don't have time to blend oils to suit my immediate need. I also may grab helichrysum essential oil in one hand and jojoba wax in the other after I stub a toe to ease the pain and prevent bruising. Generally, however, blends will serve you much better than single oils.

It's a good idea to make some "master blends" ahead of time so that you have them when you need them.

Next, let's go over some basic principles of blending and review some important safety considerations.

Principles of Blending

A great first step to understanding and identifying essential oils is learning the three categories of "notes": top notes, middle notes, and base notes (or fixatives).

Essential oils known as top notes are commonly citrus oils. Top notes are often the first noticeable aromas in a blend but also the aromas that evaporate the quickest. We could say they appear as swiftly as they depart.

Middle notes are sometimes referred to as the heart or the center of an aromatherapy blend. Their aromas will last a little longer than top notes on a perfume blotter or your skin.

The base notes are what I typically refer to as fixatives because they stick around the longest. If the oil is viscous (thick) enough, as is the case with Buddha wood, vetiver, and ruh khus, it will hold onto the middle and top notes a little bit longer.

Ideally, every blend you create should have one or more of each of these notes. Otherwise, for example, if your massage blend does not contain a base note or a fixative, the aroma will not last long at all.

Blending according to essential oil notes is not required, but the blends themselves will be balanced in aroma and therapeutics if you practice in this way. Consider Alleviate Anxiety Aromatherapy Inhaler (see page 95). This blend calls for five drops sweet orange, three drops Australian sandalwood, three drops frankincense, three drops palo santo, and one drop neroli. Adding more than three drops of neroli to this blend would overpower all the other essential oils. The same concept would apply to oils such as Roman chamomile, jasmine, or ylang-ylang.

Also, when you are ready to create your first blend, be sure to have the dilution chart (see page 30) handy. This chart will be a great reference tool for you going forward as you make the blends in this book and create ones of your own.

Layering

Whereas synergy creates a blend of oils that is greater than its parts, another technique for applying essential oils is called layering. Layering essential oils is adding oils to the skin one at a time rather than as a blend of oils in a carrier oil. Some theorize that allowing single essential oils to absorb at their own pace has certain benefits. (To learn more about this method, check out "The Complete Skin Series by Robert Tisserand" online at TisserandInstitute.org.)

Personally, I don't feel adding essential oils one at a time in this manner is harmful, but I also don't think it has an inherent benefit compared to blending. We know that the longer an essential oil stays in contact with the skin, the better the absorption. This is one reason why vegetable-based carrier oils are so important: We want the oils to stay on the skin rather than quickly evaporate. Essential oil constituents absorb into the skin at various rates based on their molecular size and structure. Whether you apply one oil or a blend, those constituents are absorbed into the bloodstream at different rates, so layering them has no real measurable or substantial advantage.

For that reason, all of the essential oils in each application or remedy in the next chapter are intended to be applied all at once, as a blend or synergy of oils.

Safety Guidelines

Before you dive into "100 Applications and Remedies" (chapter 6), please keep these safety issues in mind:

Babies and children. Some essential oils are gentle enough for babies ages 3 months and older and can be used safely on babies' skin if heavily diluted. In general, children ages 2 years and older can begin to use a longer list of essential oils topically.

Inhaler use for children. On average, the age recommendation for aromatherapy inhalers is more mature children 5 years and older. Inhalers are a direct method of inhalation, whereas diffusers are passive and more suitable for young children. Please use your discretion.

Bath oils for children. My general age recommendation for using oil in the bath with children is 5 years old and up. If your child is still putting toys in their mouth with the potential to swallow water, I recommend waiting to use oils in the bathtub.

Diffusing periods. Diffuse for 30 to 60 minutes for a healthy adult. I recommend shorter times for children, 10 to 15 minutes. To avoid overexposure, take a break after the timer goes off and the unit shuts down before turning it on again.

Pregnancy usage. As a general recommendation, essential oils should be avoided during the first trimester of pregnancy unless you are under the care of a trained aromatherapist. If you are considered high risk, you should avoid them altogether during this time.

Another consideration when making blends is knowing which oils have maximum dilution recommendations and/or photo-toxic components per the International Fragrance Association's guidelines. When you are making a blend to use on the skin in any manner, you need to get out your calculator and be sure that you are following those safety recommendations. For those oils with safety requirements in "100 Applications and Remedies" (chapter 6), I have provided blend recipes within those parameters for your safety.

CHAPTER 6

100 Applications and Remedies

You can use essential oils in a variety of ways to support emotional wellness. Many blends have been curated here for you to cover some of the most common concerns. With 100 recipes, you are sure to find something for almost every situation, including blends with fun names created just for children.

This chapter is divided into several sections, such as Anxiety, Depression, Mood, and Stress. In addition to blends featuring my top 50 essential oils for emotional wellness, you'll find a unique set of recipes for self-care and bonus blends for chakra balancing. Note that master blends can be made in larger quantities and stored for future use. Safety information also will be included as needed.

Anxiety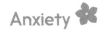

ALLEVIATE ANXIETY AROMATHERAPY INHALER

DIRECT INHALATION   Safe for Ages 5+

I carefully chose this blend of oils based on their therapeutics and the aromatic end result. Frankincense, palo santo, and sandalwood are rich, earthy, and grounding, which facilitates mood stabilization, and have a unique ability to slow down the catastrophic-type thinking that typically causes anxiety. Sweet orange essential oil has a soothing sweetness that rounds out the synergy. Use this blend to help you to find your focus when needed.

4 plastic pipettes

5 drops sweet orange essential oil

3 drops frankincense essential oil

3 drops palo santo essential oil

3 drops sandalwood essential oil

1 drop neroli essential oil

Aromatherapy inhaler

1. Using the pipettes, place the essential oils onto the cotton wick of the inhaler, and snap the cap firmly into place.

2. Carry the inhaler with you, and open the cap and inhale slowly multiple times to alleviate anxiety as needed.

BREATHE EASY AND PERSEVERE ROOM SPRAY

PASSIVE INHALATION   Safe for Ages 2+

Reach for this earthy yet light and fresh room spray when you are feeling overwhelmed, trying to release a heavy event in your past or present, or preparing to let go of deep-seated anger and need a little assistance. With its beautiful blue hue, yarrow essential oil's herbaceous scent can help you work through a traumatic experience. The combination of lime, red mandarin, and patchouli helps ground you while providing a jeweled citrus aroma. The alcohol in the recipe helps the oils dissolve in the water, stopping large oil droplets from being sprayed on linens or carpet.

3 drops yarrow essential oil

3 drops lime essential oil

3 drops patchouli essential oil

3 drops red mandarin essential oil

1 (2-ounce) glass spray bottle

½ ounce 190-proof alcohol or perfumers alcohol

Distilled water

1. Place the essential oils into the bottle.

2. Add the alcohol.

3. Fill the remainder of the bottle with distilled water.

4. Label and store in a cool place.

CLEAR AND COMPOSED FIZZY BATH BALL

TOPICAL USE   Safe for Ages 5+

This blend of essential oils imparts gentle floral and fruity notes. Relax into this aromatic bath to uplift the spirit and enjoy a deep sense of calm.

1 cup baking soda
½ cup citric acid
½ cup arrowroot powder
2 ¼ tablespoons grapeseed oil

6 drops clary sage essential oil
6 drops sweet orange essential oil

2 drops cape chamomile essential oil
¾ tablespoon distilled water

1. In a bowl, mix the baking soda, citric acid, and arrowroot powder.

2. In a separate container, blend the grapeseed oil, essential oils, and water.

3. Slowly add the wet ingredients into the dry ingredients, blending until mixed well. You can form balls using your hands, but stainless steel or silicone molds are easier and more fun.

4. Let sit to dry and harden.

5. Use one ball at a time by dropping it into the water once you are in the bath.

HAVE FAITH DIFFUSER BLEND

PASSIVE INHALATION   Safe for Ages 3+ Months

Cistus essential oil will stand out in this diffuser blend with its bright citrusy and sweet aroma, helping you have faith that everything will work out during the more challenging moments in your life. Sweet orange and bergamot orange are strong anxiolytics that help lessen situational anxiety and bring you a sense of contentment in the present. Lastly, Australian sandalwood essential oil, with its sweet and woodsy aroma, is the fixative in this blend, helping you stay grounded. This blend is sure to be a favorite.

4 drops sweet orange essential oil

2 drops bergamot orange essential oil

2 drops cistus essential oil

2 drops Australian sandalwood essential oil

Place the essential oils into your favorite diffuser according to manufacturer instructions. Use this blend as needed. Follow safe diffusing guidelines.

PEACEFUL AURA BODY OIL

TOPICAL USE   Safe for Ages 2+

Peaceful Aura is a lovely body oil, great when used right out of the shower or just before lying down for bed at night. The four oils work together in synergy to leave you in a very peaceful, contented state. If you are feeling anxious at bedtime, the cistus in this blend will go a long way to clear your head and help you sink into your body. Spikenard is calming and soothing to the heart and mind.

4 drops orange essential oil

2 drops cistus essential oil

2 drops sandalwood essential oil

1 drop spikenard essential oil

1 ounce jojoba wax

1. In a glass container, blend the essential oils into the jojoba wax.

2. Apply as needed by massaging into your skin. Store the unused portion in a cool place.

RELEASE THE FEAR DIFFUSER BLEND

PASSIVE DIFFUSION   Safe for Ages 2+

In *Aromatherapy for Healing the Spirit*, Gabriel Mojay writes that geranium can help with emotional and physical imbalances that manifest as stress, restlessness, or fear: "A combination of geranium and orange oils is called for, to pacify the will and ease frustration."[105] This synergy combines sweet orange and geranium essential oils with a small amount of sandalwood and ylang-ylang to help you to address your fears head-on.

4 drops sweet orange
essential oil

3 drops geranium
essential oil

2 drops sandalwood
essential oil

1 drop ylang-ylang
essential oil

Place the essential oils into your favorite diffuser according to manufacturer instructions. Use this blend as needed. Follow safe diffusing guidelines.

STOP OVERTHINKING AROMATHERAPY INHALER

DIRECT INHALATION   Safe for Ages 5+

This synergy aims to relieve nervous tension and allows the mind to find a sense of stillness. Petitgrain is especially helpful to slow the mind when it is on overload, and cedarwood atlas helps bring focus when you need to complete a task. If you have moments when your brain cannot stop running in all directions, reach for this aromatherapy inhaler to slow it down.

4 plastic pipettes

5 drops sandalwood essential oil

4 drops petitgrain essential oil

3 drops cedarwood atlas essential oil

3 drops lime essential oil

Aromatherapy inhaler

1. Using the pipettes, place the essential oils onto the cotton wick of the inhaler, and snap the cap firmly into place.

2. Carry the inhaler with you, and open the cap and inhale slowly multiple times to calm racing thoughts as needed.

JUST FOR CHILDREN

KISS OVERWHELM GOODBYE AROMATHERAPY INHALER

DIRECT INHALATION · Safe for Ages 5+

This blend was part of a research study published in 2012 in *Evidence-Based Complementary and Alternative Medicine*.[106] These four oils were shown to reduce blood pressure and the stress hormone cortisol in female patients, making them beneficial for situational stress and anxiety.

4 plastic pipettes
9 drops lavender essential oil

3 drops sweet marjoram essential oil
2 drops ylang-ylang essential oil

1 drop neroli essential oil
Aromatherapy inhaler

1. Using the pipettes, place the essential oils onto the cotton wick of the inhaler, and snap the cap firmly into place.

2. Carry the inhaler with you, and open the cap and inhale slowly multiple times as needed.

OH, HAPPY DAY SHOWER MELT (MASTER BLEND)

PASSIVE INHALATION   Safe for Ages 2+

A shower melt is a great alternative to an aroma bath. This one will wake you up and put a smile on your face.

5ml dark glass bottle

15 drops lemon
essential oil

10 drops grapefruit
essential oil

10 drops bergamot
orange
essential oil

5 drops black pepper
essential oil

1 cup baking soda

½ cup sea salt

2 teaspoons water

Your favorite
silicone molds

1. In the glass bottle, combine the essential oils to create a master blend. Store in a cool location until ready to use.

2. In a small bowl, mix the baking soda and sea salt.

3. Slowly add the water until you have the consistency of wet sand.

4. Press the mixture into molds to dry and set.

5. Add 5 to 7 drops of the master blend to a shower melt just before you are ready to use it.

SLOW DOWN FROWN DIFFUSER BLEND

PASSIVE INHALATION   Safe for Ages 3+ Months

Do you have a child who is not a morning person? This blend can help address the wake-up moodiness or the occasional angry outburst. Essential oils can center us enough to see the calm through the storm. This blend is warming and reassuring with a resinous, floral aroma and citrus undertones. The hippies of the 1960s were onto something with patchouli, and artfully blending it with sweet orange and neroli makes a synergy that is truly divine.

6 drops sweet orange
    essential oil
2 drops patchouli
    essential oil

1 drop balsam copaiba
    essential oil
1 drop neroli
    essential oil

Place the essential oils into your favorite diffuser according to manufacturer instructions. Use this blend as needed. Follow safe diffusing guidelines.

Depression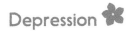

BRIGHT AND BLISSFUL ANOINTING OIL

TOPICAL USE   Safe for Ages 2+

Although these oils are safe for children ages 2 and older, this particular blend is intended for adults. The combination of sensual and radiant davana with the sweetness of orange and bright floral undertones makes this blend supportive during times of situational anxiety and depression.

3 drops davana
    essential oil

3 drops sweet orange
    essential oil

2 drops clary sage
    essential oil

1 drop rhododendron
    essential oil

1 ounce jojoba wax

1. In a glass container, blend the essential oils into the jojoba wax.

2. Apply as needed, anointing your chakras or massaging into skin as a moisturizing blend. Store the unused portion in a cool place.

CHEERFUL CITRUS AROMATHERAPY INHALER

DIRECT INHALATION   Safe for Ages 5+

It is all citrus on board for this cheerful aromatherapy inhaler blend, and everyone in the family is sure to love it. Gray days, not enough sleep, or feeling moody—all are good reasons to reach for this inhaler synergy to cheer you right up. Alternatively, you can place this blend in your favorite diffuser and fill the home with good vibes.

4 plastic pipettes

5 drops lemon essential oil

4 drops bergamot orange essential oil

3 drops red mandarin essential oil

3 drops sweet orange essential oil

1 aromatherapy inhaler

1. Using the pipettes, place the essential oils onto the cotton wick of the inhaler, and snap the cap firmly into place.

2. Carry the inhaler with you, and open the cap and inhale slowly multiple times to perk up your mood as needed.

FINDING SOLACE DIFFUSER BLEND (MASTER BLEND)

PASSIVE INHALATION   Safe for Ages 3+ Months

Australian sandalwood and vetiver essential oils are self-nourishing and comforting, helping settle irritability and agitation. Added to these two mental wellness powerhouses are red mandarin and jasmine for times of vulnerability and fragility, providing you solace and hope. Red mandarin reminds you of the importance of self-care. Place this synergy in your diffuser to help increase confidence and promote positive thinking.

5ml dark glass bottle
20 drops red mandarin essential oil

10 drops Australian sandalwood essential oil

6 drops vetiver essential oil
4 drops jasmine essential oil

1. In the glass bottle, combine the essential oils to create a master blend. Store in a cool location until ready to use.

2. Add as desired to your favorite diffuser according to manufacturer instructions. Follow safe diffusing guidelines.

INSPIRING HOPE BATH SALTS (MASTER BLEND)

TOPICAL USE   Safe for Ages 5+

The essential oils in this blend are safe for children ages 5 years and up, but this synergy is geared toward older children and adults. This blend is intended to renew faith in your life situation, helping you be more optimistic while strengthening your nervous system. Black spruce is integral to the support and balance of our endocrine system, according to aromatherapy pioneer Kurt Schnaubelt.[107] If you are beginning to feel burned out, add black spruce to your daily wellness routine.

5ml dark glass bottle

15 drops lavender
essential oil

10 drops clary sage
essential oil

8 drops myrrh
essential oil

7 drops black spruce
essential oil

1 tablespoon
carrier oil

1 cup Epsom salts
(optional)

½ cup full-fat
coconut cream
(optional)

1. In the glass bottle, combine the essential oils to create a master blend. Store in a cool location until ready to use.

2. Mix 5 to 7 drops of the master blend with the carrier oil, and add to the Epsom salts, if using, or directly to the bathwater. If using the coconut cream, add it to the bathwater last.

RELEASE THE ANGER AROMATHERAPY INHALER

DIRECT INHALATION   Safe for Ages 5+

Bergamot orange is the primary essential oil used in this inhalation
blend for its ability to relieve the mind of mental and emotional
fatigue caused by anger, confusion, and stress. The combination of
cistus, rose otto, and ruh khus helps promote calm and centered-
ness during or after an emotional event or upheaval. When you
are feeling angry or as if the world has handed you more than
you can handle, reach for this synergy to begin working through
your feelings.

4 plastic pipettes	3 drops cistus	2 drops ruh khus
8 drops bergamot	essential oil	essential oil
orange	2 drops rose otto	Aromatherapy
essential oil	essential oil	inhaler

1. Using the pipettes, place the essential oils onto the cotton wick
   of the inhaler, and snap the cap firmly into place.

2. Carry the inhaler with you, and open the cap and inhale slowly
   multiple times as needed.

SOFTEN THE HEART BODY OIL

TOPICAL USE   Safe for Ages 2+

The comforting and grounding aspects of frankincense and myrrh essential oils calm and settle the heart, bringing a sense of balance to troubled times. Spikenard is an intentional addition to this synergy to assist in releasing the past. Rose otto opens the heart, removing self-doubt and judgment and helping foster feelings self-love and forgiveness.

3 drops frankincense essential oil

2 drops myrrh essential oil

2 drops rose otto essential oil

2 drops spikenard essential oil

1 drop lime essential oil

1 ounce jojoba wax

1. In a glass container, blend the essential oils into the jojoba wax.

2. Apply as needed, anointing your chakras or massaging into skin as a moisturizing blend. Store the unused portion in a cool place.

THE SUN WILL COME OUT DIFFUSER BLEND

This synergy has a unique aroma: herbaceous, peppery, and citrusy with a heady floral hint. Sweet orange and blue tansy blend quite well together, and pink pepper adds a refreshing addition to the blend. Jasmine essential oil, when added in a small amount, is uplifting and transformative without being overwhelming. I dare you to not smile after sitting with this blend for a while.

5 drops sweet orange
    essential oil
2 drops blue tansy
    essential oil

2 drops pink pepper
    essential oil
1 drop jasmine
    essential oil

Place the essential oils into your favorite diffuser according to manufacturer instructions. Use this blend as needed. Follow safe diffusing guidelines.

JUST FOR CHILDREN

BE HOPEFUL ROLLERBALL BLEND (MASTER BLEND)

TOPICAL USE   Safe for Ages 2+

Your children will adore this blend made especially for them. It is a sublime combination of refreshing and uplifting citrus essential oils. This synergy can restore anyone's outlook on a dreary, cloudy day.

5ml dark glass bottle
1 plastic pipette
10 drops lemon
    essential oil
5 drops davana
    essential oil
5 drops grapefruit
    essential oil

5 drops lavender
    essential oil
5 drops lime
    essential oil
5 drops red mandarin
    essential oil
5 drops sweet orange
    essential oil

10ml amber or
    cobalt glass
    rollerball bottle
~9ml carrier oil

1. In the glass bottle, combine the essential oils to create a master blend. Store in a cool location until ready for use.

2. Add 6 drops of master blend to the rollerball bottle.

3. Fill the remainder of the bottle with the carrier oil, leaving enough space at the top for the rollerball applicator so your oils do not overflow.

4. Pop in the rollerball applicator, and cap tightly.

5. Apply topically as needed.

HAVE FAITH AROMATHERAPY INHALER

DIRECT INHALATION   Safe for Ages 5+

This essential oil blend is formulated specifically for children in mind. When your child is going through a tough time, whether it's due to stress, anxiety, or situational depression, this blend will be a great aid. With this aromatherapy inhaler, you can comfort them while they breathe in the healing synergy. With your help, they'll know that everything is going to be okay.

4 plastic pipettes

6 drops red mandarin essential oil

6 drops sweet orange essential oil

2 drops sandalwood essential oil

1 drop ylang-ylang essential oil

Aromatherapy inhaler

1. Using the pipettes, place the essential oils onto the cotton wick of the inhaler, and snap the cap firmly into place.

2. Carry the inhaler with you, and open the cap and inhale slowly multiple times as needed.

LET IT ALL GO BATH BLEND (MASTER BLEND)

TOPICAL USE   Safe for Ages 5+

Your children will love this bath blend. It has everything needed to wind down at the end of a busy, hectic day to ensure a restorative night's sleep. Bergamot mint, lavender, and neroli are powerhouse sedative, feel-good oils. The small amount of rose in this master blend rounds out the aroma quite nicely but is not overpowering.

5ml dark glass bottle

20 drops bergamot mint essential oil

10 drops lavender essential oil

7 drops neroli essential oil

3 drops rose otto essential oil

1 tablespoon carrier oil

1 cup Epsom salts (optional)

½ cup full-fat coconut cream (optional)

1. In the glass bottle, combine the essential oils to create a master blend. Store in a cool location until ready to use.

2. Mix 5 to 7 drops of the master blend with the carrier oil, and add to the Epsom salts, if using, or directly to the bathwater. If using the coconut cream, add it to the bathwater last.

Mood

BRIGHT AND CHEERFUL DIFFUSER BLEND

PASSIVE INHALATION   Safe for Ages 3+ Months

The bright and cheery citrus aroma of grapefruit combined with the floral undertones of petitgrain and ylang-ylang is perfect for when you are feeling irritable or grumpy and need a bit of an emotional adjustment. Put up your feet with this trio, and feel your mood quickly begin to shift.

| 6 drops grapefruit | 2 drops petitgrain | 2 drops ylang-ylang |
| essential oil | essential oil | essential oil |

Place the essential oils into your favorite diffuser according to manufacturer instructions. Use this blend as needed. Follow safe diffusing guidelines.

CLEAR THE ENERGY ROOM SPRAY

Buddha wood is the highlight in this essential oil room spray that helps you clear energy in the home. When combined with elemi, sweet orange, and frankincense essential oils, it imparts a woody, spicy aroma with citrusy-sweet undertones. Try this room spray while journaling about what you're ready to let go, and feel the energy shift.

5 drops sweet orange essential oil

3 drops elemi essential oil

3 drops Buddha wood essential oil

1 drop frankincense essential oil

1 (2-ounce) glass spray bottle

½ ounce 190-proof alcohol or perfumers alcohol

Distilled water

1. Place the essential oils into the bottle.

2. Add the alcohol to help the oils dissolve.

3. Fill the remainder of the bottle with distilled water.

4. Label and store in a cool place.

FIND YOUR ENTHUSIASM DIFFUSER BLEND

PASSIVE INHALATION   Safe for Ages 3+ Months

This lively, energizing blend of essential oils is sure to get you out of a rut in no time flat. Sweet basil is invigorating, providing mental focus and vigor. When combined with lemon and Siberian fir, it opens your airways, clears your mind, and leaves you renewed and ready to take on the day. Plus, if friends visit after this zesty aroma has been diffused, they're sure to think you just cleaned your home.

4 drops sweet basil   3 drops lemon   3 drops Siberian fir
essential oil   essential oil   essential oil

Place the essential oils into your favorite diffuser according to manufacturer instructions. Use this blend as needed. Follow safe diffusing guidelines.

GOOD SPIRITS AROMATHERAPY INHALER

DIRECT INHALATION   Safe for Ages 5+

The zesty, citrusy blend of elemi, lemon, and red mandarin essential oils will put you in good spirits when you need a quick attitude change. Ylang-ylang adds a heady floral scent that uplifts the mood and reduces anxiety to provide calm. Sandalwood is a fixative that helps pull down the other oils in the blend, reducing any agitation and unease while providing you a sense of serenity and contentment.

5 plastic pipettes

5 drops lemon
essential oil

3 drops red mandarin
essential oil

3 drops sandalwood
essential oil

2 drops elemi
essential oil

2 drops ylang-ylang
essential oil

Aromatherapy
inhaler

1. Using the pipettes, place the essential oils onto the cotton wick of the inhaler, and snap the cap firmly into place.

2. Carry the inhaler with you, and open the cap and inhale slowly multiple times as needed.

HAPPINESS GUARANTEED DIFFUSER BLEND

DIRECT INHALATION   Safe for Ages 3+ Months

This combination of essential oil goodness will put your hectic schedule behind you and pave the way for some rest and relaxation when you are done with the day and need some emotional relief.

5 drops lime
    essential oil
2 drops black pepper
    essential oil

2 drops bergamot
    orange
    essential oil

1 drop cypress
    essential oil

Place the essential oils into your favorite diffuser according to manufacturer instructions. Use this blend as needed. Follow safe diffusing guidelines.

REFRESHED AND ALERT AROMATHERAPY INHALER

DIRECT INHALATION   Safe for Ages 5+

This blend of zesty black pepper and lime will leave you feeling revitalized. Cypress essential oil, with its fresh and green aroma, complements it nicely, helping open your airways and wake you up. Lastly, bergamot orange essential oil helps soften the blend and adds the perfect amount of citrus. Carry this portable inhaler with you if you suffer from an afternoon slump. It also can help stop food cravings triggered by emotions.

4 plastic pipettes

6 drops lime
  essential oil

4 drops black pepper
  essential oil

3 drops bergamot
  orange
  essential oil

2 drops cypress
  essential oil

Aromatherapy
  inhaler

1. Using the pipettes, place the essential oils onto the cotton wick of the inhaler, and snap the cap firmly into place.

2. Carry the inhaler with you, and open the cap and inhale slowly multiple times as needed.

WAKE UP SHOWER MELTS (MASTER BLEND)

PASSIVE INHALATION   Safe for Ages 2+

Do you struggle with the morning routine? Do you suffer from chronic stress, or are you feeling burned out? Start the morning with the energizing, uplifting aroma of sweet basil, which is one of my first recommendations for anyone who needs to stay on task and wants help with memory retention. This blend is balanced out with lemon and lime and is guaranteed to provide a stimulating shower experience.

5ml dark glass bottle

15 drops sweet basil essential oil

15 drops lemon essential oil

15 drops lime essential oil

1 cup baking soda

½ cup sea salt

2 teaspoons distilled water

Your favorite silicone molds

1. In the glass bottle, combine the essential oils to create a master blend. Store in a cool location until ready to use.

2. In a small bowl, mix the baking soda and salt. Slowly add the water until you have the consistency of wet sand.

3. Press the mixture into molds to dry and set.

4. Add 5 to 7 drops of the master blend to a shower melt just before you are ready to use it. Store the bottle containing any unused master blend in a cool place.

JUST FOR CHILDREN

GRUMPY GUS DIFFUSER BLEND

PASSIVE INHALATION   Safe for Ages 3+ Months

This essential oil synergy is formulated especially for your children. We are not strangers to their irritable moods, and they can use some emotional assistance when they have a hard time expressing what they are feeling, are overstimulated, or are just plain tired. Kids will love the aroma of this citrus blend with a bit of grounding from frankincense. Put these oils in their favorite diffuser to ease the whining and have them smiling once again.

4 drops lime essential oil

3 drops lemon essential oil

2 drops frankincense essential oil

1 drop sweet orange essential oil

Place the essential oils into your favorite diffuser according to manufacturer instructions. Use this blend as needed. Follow safe diffusing guidelines, and when it comes to children, remember that less is more.

TAME TEMPER MASSAGE OIL

TOPICAL USE   Safe for Ages 2+

Nothing is quite like a parent's touch when children are over-stimulated and restless. This massage oil provides a heavenly blend of oils that will have them feeling serene in mere minutes. The esters in clary sage, the floral deliciousness of jasmine, and the purifying aspects of frankincense, myrrh, and patchouli make this synergy a sure winner. Try putting this blend in a diffuser if your child is not in a headspace to be touched, and don't be shy about using this blend yourself.

3 drops clary sage essential oil

3 drops frankincense essential oil

1 drop jasmine essential oil

1 drop myrrh essential oil

1 drop patchouli essential oil

1 ounce grapeseed oil

1. Combine all the oils in a glass container.

2. Massage into your child's arms, chest, and legs. Use as needed. Store unused portion in a cool place.

WIPE THEIR TEARS ROLLERBALL BLEND

TOPICAL USE   Safe for Ages 2+

This blend, formulated especially for a child, has a lovely warm, radiant, woody, and sweet aroma with citrus and floral undertones. Even in minute amounts, palo santo ushers in calm and helps foster peace. If your child is dealing with low self-esteem or self-worth due to teasing or bullying, use this blend near the nose for maximum inhalation.

1 plastic pipette	2 drops petitgrain essential oil	10ml amber or cobalt glass
3 drops lime essential oil	1 drop palo santo essential oil	rollerball bottle
		~9ml carrier oil

1. Using the pipette, add the essential oils to the rollerball bottle.

2. Fill the remainder of the bottle with the carrier oil, leaving enough space at the top for the rollerball applicator so your oils do not overflow.

3. Pop in the rollerball applicator, and cap tightly.

4. Apply topically as needed.

Stress

BLISSED PERSONAL PERFUME

TOPICAL USE   Safe for Ages 2+

This perfume blend is safe around children but is intended for adults. Its unique blend of oils in a base of vanilla-infused jojoba wax is truly divine. When I apply this synergy before leaving the house for the day, I prepare myself for the attention I attract. Ylang-ylang can be overwhelming for some people, but it's virtually unnoticeable in this artfully blended perfume.

3 drops davana essential oil

3 drops red mandarin essential oil

1 drop sandalwood essential oil

1 drop ylang-ylang essential oil

9 drops plain or vanilla-infused jojoba wax (see Tip)

1. In a glass container, blend the essential oils into the jojoba wax.

2. Apply to points on neck and wrists, massaging into your skin. Store unused portion in a cool place.

Tip: Infusing your own vanilla beans in jojoba wax is easy and economical, and the vanilla will help the essential oils remain on the skin longer. Halve 2 vanilla beans lengthwise and cut into small pieces. Place in a clear glass jar, cover with 1 cup jojoba wax, and cap. Store in a warm spot, shaking periodically, for a minimum of 4 weeks. Strain the beans using cheese-cloth, and pour your vanilla-infused jojoba wax into a separate bottle to store.

BREAK FROM THE TENSION DIFFUSER BLEND

PASSIVE INHALATION   Safe for Ages 3+ Months

When we reach for blue tansy essential oil, we tend to think about how it helps us with seasonal allergies or supports a healthy respiratory system, but blue tansy also is beneficial for soothing stress and anxiety. This deep blue oil blends nicely with clary sage, lavender, and petitgrain, helping take the bite out of the herbaceous aroma of blue tansy while enhancing its therapeutic effects. The aroma of this diffuser blend is heavenly and effective when you need emotional nourishing.

4 drops clary sage
    essential oil
3 drops lavender
    essential oil

2 drops blue tansy
    essential oil
1 drop petitgrain
    essential oil

Place the essential oils into your favorite diffuser according to manufacturer instructions. Use this blend as needed. Follow safe diffusing guidelines, and when it comes to children, remember that less is more.

CALMING THE NERVES DIFFUSER BLEND (MASTER BLEND)

PASSIVE INHALATION   Safe for Ages 3+ Months

This blend is perhaps my favorite calming blend for the home. I always keep a master blend bottled and ready for use. It has seen diffusers, inhalers, even a teddy bear or two. The synergy of sedatives cannot be beat. When you are feeling frayed and burned out, place this blend of oils in your diffuser, and allow yourself to truly relax and let go.

5ml dark glass bottle
10 drops lavandin essential oil
10 drops patchouli essential oil

10 drops red mandarin essential oil
5 drops cape chamomile essential oil

5 drops neroli essential oil

1. In the glass bottle, combine the essential oils to create a master blend. Store in a cool location until ready to use.

2. Add as desired to your favorite diffuser according to manufacturer instructions. Follow safe diffusing guidelines.

RELEASE THE PRESSURE AROMATHERAPY INHALER

DIRECT INHALATION   Safe for Ages 5+

When you're feeling overwhelmed, reach for the following blend of essential oils to restore tranquility and harmony with body, mind, and spirit. The synergy of red mandarin, lavender, and Australian sandalwood ushers in peace and emotional fortitude. One drop of angelica root rounds out this blend to help rebuild your strength to get through any tough situation with grace. It's recommended for inhalation over topical use due to the photo-sensitizing quality of angelica root, which requires caution.

4 plastic pipettes	3 drops Australian sandalwood essential oil	Aromatherapy inhaler
7 drops red mandarin essential oil		
4 drops lavender essential oil	1 drop angelica root essential oil	

1. Using the pipettes, place the essential oils onto the cotton wick of the inhaler, and snap the cap firmly into place.

2. Carry the inhaler with you, and open the cap and inhale slowly multiple times as needed.

REST EASY BATH SALTS (MASTER BLEND)

TOPICAL USE   Safe for Ages 5+

Are you looking to unwind at the end of a hectic day? Self-care is incredibly important for all of us, but even more so when we are feeling stressed out. The use of Epsom salts in the bath with this heavenly synergy will quiet your mind and settle your parasympathetic nervous system. It's important to make sure that you are diluting your oils properly in the bath to lower the risk of skin irritation, especially for more sensitive skin.

5ml dark glass bottle
15 drops red mandarin essential oil
15 drops sweet orange essential oil

5 drops myrrh essential oil
5 drops vetiver essential oil
1 tablespoon carrier oil

1 cup Epsom salts (optional)
½ cup full-fat coconut cream (optional)

1. In the glass bottle, combine the essential oils to create a master blend. Store in a cool location until ready to use.

2. Mix 5 to 7 drops of the master blend with the carrier oil, and add to the Epsom salts, if using, or directly to bathwater. If using the coconut cream, add it to the bathwater last.

RESTORE TRANQUILITY AROMATHERAPY INHALER

DIRECT INHALATION   Safe for Ages 5+

This synergy is formulated for teens and women with symptoms of PMS. Clary sage is a powerhouse for PMS and addresses moodiness, headaches, and even cramping quite well. Geranium essential oil also has been shown in studies to benefit PMS through massage, but inhalation is equally effective.[108] The combination of davana, ylang-ylang, and patchouli oils increases calm when you need it the most.

5 plastic pipettes

5 drops clary sage essential oil

5 drops geranium essential oil

2 drops davana essential oil

2 drops ylang-ylang essential oil

1 drop patchouli essential oil

Aromatherapy inhaler

1. Using the pipettes, place the essential oils onto the cotton wick of the inhaler, and snap the cap firmly into place.

2. Carry the inhaler with you, and open the cap and inhale slowly multiple times as needed.

REJUVENATION DIFFUSER BLEND (MASTER BLEND)

PASSIVE INHALATION   Safe for Ages 2+

Galbanum has a strong aromatic profile along with an equally strong affinity to the nervous system, especially when used with black spruce.[109] Laurel leaf was chosen for its bright profile and its ability to help you be more positive. Cypress is helpful for overwhelming transitions in life, such as a new job, a move, divorce, illness, and so on. Lastly, orange essential oil, the universal oil, rounds out this rejuvenation blend.

5ml dark glass bottle

12 drops sweet orange essential oil

10 drops laurel leaf essential oil

8 drops black spruce essential oil

6 drops cypress essential oil

4 drops galbanum essential oil

1. In the glass bottle, combine the essential oils to create a master blend. Store in a cool location until ready to use.

2. Add as desired to your favorite diffuser according to manufacturer instructions. Follow safe diffusing guidelines.

JUST FOR CHILDREN

MONSTER AWAY ROOM SPRAY

PASSIVE INHALATION   Safe for Ages 2+

Most children have times in their lives when they fear to go to sleep due to separation anxiety or a fear of monsters under the bed or in the closet. This essential oil spray is rich in child-friendly calming and reassuring essential oils. Each one of the oils in this blend has gentle sedative properties, so spraying this blend into the air and over linens will quickly result in a happy, sleeping child.

3 drops sweet marjoram essential oil

3 drops sweet orange essential oil

2 drops cedarwood atlas essential oil

2 drops lavender essential oil

1 drop cistus essential oil

1 drop vetiver essential oil

1 (2-ounce) glass spray bottle

½ ounce 190-proof alcohol or perfumers alcohol

Distilled water

1. Place the essential oils into the bottle.

2. Add the alcohol to help the oils dissolve.

3. Fill the remainder of the bottle with distilled water.

4. Label and store in a cool place.

PEACEFUL TOTS BEDTIME BATH BLEND

TOPICAL USE   Safe for Ages 5+

Schedules are always busy, and even our children are not immune to the stress. School, homework, sports, and other events can leave children wound up at the end of the day and unwilling to go to bed or, worse, unable to fall asleep. If this sounds familiar, a bath time ritual may be your answer to a smoother bedtime routine.

3 drops cape chamomile essential oil

1 drop ho wood essential oil

1 drop sweet marjoram essential oil

1 drop sweet orange essential oil

1 tablespoon carrier oil

½ cup Epsom salts (optional)

1. Mix the essential oils into your carrier oil, and add to the Epsom salts, if using, or directly to the bathwater.

2. If your child is young, make sure you explain that they are not to swallow water, dunk their head, or open their eyes underwater, all of which can increase the risk of irritation. Always supervise children in the bathtub.

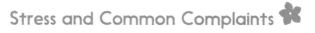

ACHES AND PAINS

MUSCLE CALM MASSAGE OIL

TOPICAL USE   Safe for Ages 2+

Although these essential oils are safe topically for children ages 2 years and up, this massage oil is geared toward older children and adults. The synergistic blend of oils helps quell inflammation and greatly reduce aches and pains in muscles and joints. This blend is a 1 percent dilution of essential oils to carrier oil, but you may find that 2 to 3 percent may be more effective on concentrated areas of the body. This blend can be used at 3 percent dilution without risk of skin irritation.

3 drops balsam copaiba essential oil

2 drops black pepper essential oil

2 drops hemp essential oil

1 drop helichrysum essential oil

1 drop Roman chamomile

1 ounce jojoba wax

1. In a glass container, blend the essential oils into the jojoba wax.

2. Apply to trouble areas as needed. Store the unused portion in a cool place.

SOOTHING BATH SALTS (MASTER BLEND)

TOPICAL USE   Safe for Ages 5+

This synergy is geared toward older children and adults, especially those who adore an aromatic bath when their body aches. My aches and pains increase with my stress levels, and this synergy has provided incredibly effective relief.

5ml dark glass bottle
20 drops lavandin
    essential oil
10 drops helichrysum
    essential oil

5 drops Australian
    sandalwood
    essential oil
5 drops balsam
    copaiba
    essential oil

1 tablespoon
    grapeseed oil
1 cup Epsom salts
¼ cup baking soda
¼ cup pink Himalayan
    sea salt

1. In the glass bottle, combine the essential oils to create a master blend. Store in a cool location until ready to use.

2. In a small bowl, pour in the grapeseed oil.

3. Mix 5 to 7 drops of the master blend into the grapeseed oil.

4. In a medium bowl, mix the Epsom salts, baking soda, and Himalayan sea salt.

5. Add the oils to the dry ingredients, mixing well.

6. Add the blend to the bath, and enjoy.

STRESS ACHE BODY OIL

TOPICAL USE   Safe for Ages 5+

Massage this synergy of essential oils into your child's legs when they are experiencing growing pains or muscle fatigue from sports or general overexertion. Sweet marjoram helps address muscle spasms, and blue tansy is an anti-inflammatory with a scent adored by children and adults. Spikenard is included in this blend based solely on personal experience. My stress sits in my shoulders and neck, and spikenard works hard at softening those muscles while easing my mind.

3 drops sweet marjoram essential oil

2 drops Australian sandalwood essential oil

2 drops sweet orange essential oil

1 drop blue tansy essential oil

1 drop spikenard essential oil

1 ounce jojoba wax

1. In a glass container, blend the essential oils into the jojoba wax.

2. Apply to trouble areas as needed. Store the unused portion in a cool place.

CHANGES IN APPETITE

PASSIVE INHALATION   Safe for Ages 3+ Months

We are all under stress, and the effects of that stress can differ from person to person. Some of us lose our appetite, but many of us find ourselves with food cravings or eat when we're not hungry. Emotional eating is common, and essential oils can help combat it. Next time you are thinking of reaching for that extra snack, turn on your diffuser instead.

3 drops bergamot orange essential oil

3 drops lavender essential oil

2 drops clary sage essential oil

2 drops frankincense essential oil

Place the essential oils into your favorite diffuser according to manufacturer instructions. Follow safe diffusing guidelines. Alternatively, you can adjust the number of drops for an on-the-go aromatherapy inhaler.

INCREASE THE APPETITE AROMATHERAPY INHALER

DIRECT INHALATION   Safe for Ages 5+

Lack of appetite can happen when we are dealing with situational anxiety and depression as well as during times of illness or convalescence. Cardamom essential oil bears many uses in aromatherapy, including helping stimulate our appetite. The juicy aroma of sweet orange helps calm both the mind and the belly, making eating seem more doable. Roman chamomile has been used traditionally to calm an upset stomach, strengthen digestion, and support the appetite. The synergy of these three essential oils is evident when we are looking to eat a healthy, comforting meal.

3 plastic pipettes	6 drops sweet orange essential oil	Aromatherapy inhaler
7 drops cardamom essential oil	2 drops Roman chamomile essential oil	

1. Using the pipettes, place the essential oils onto the cotton wick of the inhaler, and snap the cap firmly into place.

2. Carry the inhaler with you, and open the cap and inhale slowly multiple times as needed.

STOP THE CRAVINGS AROMATHERAPY INHALER

DIRECT INHALATION   Safe for Ages 5+

It's common to have food cravings when we're under stress or feeling angry or depressed, and research shows that grapefruit oil is a powerful appetite suppressant.[110] Grapefruit can help you lose weight by slowing down the craving for unhealthy sugary foods. Bergamot orange, balsam copaiba, and ylang-ylang also assist in addressing the emotions that beckon you to the refrigerator or pantry.

4 plastic pipettes
8 drops grapefruit
    essential oil
3 drops bergamot
    orange
    essential oil

3 drops balsam
    copaiba
    essential oil
1 drop ylang-ylang
    essential oil

Aromatherapy
    inhaler

1. Using the pipettes, place the essential oils onto the cotton wick of the inhaler, and snap the cap firmly into place.

2. Carry the inhaler with you, and open the cap and inhale slowly multiple times as needed.

Digestive Woes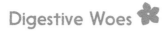

ATE TOO MUCH BELLY OIL

DIRECT INHALATION

Safe for Ages 2+
Keep away from the face of
a young child (under 10)

We all have moments of either eating too much or eating something that doesn't agree with our belly. Essential oils are powerful in this regard. Many essential oils can assist in digesting food, reducing cramping and gas, eliminating heartburn, and easing constipation. This blend of essential oils covers much of the discomfort that can arise from indulging a bit too much during a meal.

3 drops cardamom essential oil

3 drops laurel leaf essential oil

2 drops bergamot orange essential oil

1 drop Roman chamomile essential oil

1 ounce jojoba wax

1. In a glass container, blend the essential oils into the jojoba wax.

2. Apply to the belly in a clockwise, circular motion, beginning on your right side. Use a heat pack, too, if desired.

DIGESTIVE FIRE BELLY OIL

TOPICAL USE   Safe for Ages 2+
                        Keep away from the face of
                         a young child (under 10)

This blend is similar to Ate Too Much Belly Oil (see page 140) but with a stronger warming effect. When you are feeling miserable from something that did not agree with your stomach, the warmth of black pepper with cardamom is soothing and comforting. Roman chamomile can help with gas and cramping associated with food poisoning. Sweet orange helps stimulate digestion while soothing your belly and your mind.

3 drops black pepper essential oil

3 drops cardamom essential oil

2 drops sweet orange essential oil

1 drop Roman chamomile essential oil

1 ounce jojoba wax

1. In a glass container, blend the essential oils into the jojoba wax.

2. Apply to the belly in a clockwise, circular motion, beginning on your right side. Use a warm compress or heating pad, if desired.

LISTEN TO YOUR GUT AROMATHERAPY INHALER

DIRECT INHALATION   Safe for Ages 5+

My son and I react to short-term stress with upset stomachs and queasiness. Not all stomach blends aid in digestion, so this one was formulated with specifically that treatment in mind. In this blend are two stomach-supportive oils along with two stress-supportive oils. At the first sign of stomach upset, sit in a comfortable seated position focusing solely on your breath with this inhaler under your nose.

4 plastic pipettes

6 drops bergamot mint essential oil

4 drops red mandarin essential oil

3 drops Roman chamomile essential oil

2 drops vetiver essential oil

Aromatherapy inhaler

1. Using the pipettes, place the essential oils onto the cotton wick of the inhaler, and snap the cap firmly into place.

2. Carry the inhaler with you, and open the cap and inhale slowly multiple times as needed.

JUST FOR CHILDREN

BELLY BLUES BANISHED BELLY OIL

TOPICAL USE   Safe for Ages 2+

This blend was specially formulated for little bellies. Upset stomachs are common in little children when food intolerances have yet to be discovered or constipation wreaks havoc. Older children also can have stomach upset due to stress and anxiety. This belly-soothing blend has been a blessing for my boys, and I know it will be for your children, too. Rub into the lower abdomen to calm the belly, settle gas pains, help facilitate elimination, and soothe the nervous system via inhalation.

3 drops sweet
    marjoram
    essential oil
2 drops lavender
    essential oil

2 drops Roman
    chamomile
    essential oil

2 drops sweet orange
    essential oil
1 ounce grapeseed oil

1. Blend the essential oils with the grapeseed oil.

2. Apply to the belly in a clockwise, circular motion, beginning on your right side. Use a warm compress or heating pad, if desired.

RUMBLE GRUMBLE ROLLERBALL BLEND

TOPICAL USE   Safe for Ages 2+

This blend was specially formulated for little bellies on the go.
I am fond of keeping a kind of essential oils first-aid kit handy
when we are away from home, especially when we go out to eat.
If one of my children complains of belly pain from overeating,
heartburn, or indigestion, we don't need to wait until we get
home to treat it.

1 plastic pipette

2 drops sweet basil essential oil

2 drops sweet orange essential oil

1 drop red mandarin essential oil

1 drop petitgrain essential oil

10ml amber or cobalt glass rollerball bottle

~9ml carrier oil

1. Using the pipette, add the essential oils to the rollerball bottle.

2. Fill the remainder of the bottle with the carrier oil, leaving enough space at the top for the rollerball applicator so your oils do not overflow.

3. Pop in the rollerball applicator, and cap tightly.

4. Apply topically as needed.

Focus Blends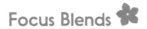

DIRECT INHALATION   Safe for Ages 5+

Whether it's due to stress or anxiety, sleepless nights, brain fog, or attention deficit/hyperactivity disorder, individuals who struggle with concentration and focus know how serious and incredibly frustrating it can be. Essential oils aid in the moment, but sometimes it takes a little bit of blending to see if they work for you. This blend is helpful for many people, and it smells amazing, too.

3 plastic pipettes	5 drops sweet basil	Aromatherapy
7 drops lime	essential oil	inhaler
essential oil	3 drops vetiver	
	essential oil	

1. Using the pipettes, place the essential oils onto the cotton wick of the inhaler, and snap the cap firmly into place.

2. Carry the inhaler with you, and open the cap and inhale multiple times to get focused before you tackle your goals.

GROUNDING ROLLERBALL BLEND

TOPICAL USE   Safe for Ages 2+

Although these essential oils are safe topically for children ages 2 and up, this rollerball synergy is geared toward older kids and adults at a slightly higher dilution rate of 3 percent. The synergy of these essential oils provides deep grounding, like the roots of a tree, so you can achieve great focus.

1 plastic pipette

4 drops cypress essential oil

2 drops cape chamomile essential oil

2 drops cedarwood atlas essential oil

1 drop palo santo essential oil

10ml amber or cobalt glass rollerball bottle

~9ml carrier oil

1. Using the pipette, add the essential oils to the rollerball bottle.

2. Fill the remainder of the bottle with the carrier oil, leaving enough space at the top for the rollerball applicator so your oils do not overflow.

3. Pop in the rollerball applicator, and cap tightly.

4. Apply topically as needed.

SQUIRRELY BRAIN DIFFUSER BLEND

Squirrely Brain is the last of the three blends I recommend for concentration and focus for all ages, and it's just as effective as the others. Petitgrain is a powerful ally to stop the brain from running on fast-forward, or with too many "tabs" open. Petitgrain and cypress together assist in slowing down thoughts. The addition of lime and grapefruit helps energize and clear the energy field, open the sinuses, and carry more oxygen to the brain so you can get your work done.

4 drops lime
    essential oil
3 drops grapefruit
    essential oil

2 drops petitgrain
    essential oil
1 drop cypress
    essential oil

Place the essential oils into your favorite diffuser according to manufacturer instructions. Use this blend as needed. Follow safe diffusing guidelines.

JUST FOR CHILDREN

HOMEWORK TIME DIFFUSER BLEND

PASSIVE INHALATION   Safe for Ages 3+ Months

This essential oil blend is perfect if you regularly struggle with your children over doing homework. It can help them focus and reduce their frustration when they sit down to work. Vetiver is the classic essential oil recommended for focus because it's effective. This synergy of oils, each with its own strengths, makes for a very efficacious blend.

4 drops lime
    essential oil
2 drops lavender
    essential oil

2 drops pink pepper
    essential oil
1 drop petitgrain
    essential oil

1 drop vetiver
    essential oil

Place the essential oils into your favorite diffuser according to manufacturer instructions. Use this blend as needed. Follow safe diffusing guidelines.

Headache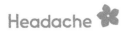

PRESSURE RELEASE MASSAGE OIL

TOPICAL USE   Safe for Ages 2+

Headaches can be tough to address with essential oils if the cause is unknown. This particular synergy is for headaches due to tension and stress. Massaging this blend of essential oils into the neck and shoulders soothes tight muscles and tension headaches. If you hold stress in your shoulders or have poor posture, this massage oil will prove very helpful for you.

4 drops lavender essential oil

2 drops sweet marjoram essential oil

2 drops sweet basil essential oil

1 drop Roman chamomile essential oil

1 ounce jojoba wax

1. In a glass container, blend the essential oils into the jojoba wax.

2. Massage into your shoulders and neck, following up with a warm compress or heating pad. Use as needed. Store unused portion in a cool place.

RELEASE THE TENSION ROLLERBALL BLEND

TOPICAL USE   Safe for Ages 2+

Although the oils in this blend are safe for children ages 2 years and older, this rollerball blend is specifically formulated for adults at a higher dilution rate of 3 percent. This particular synergy addresses headaches due to tension as well as headaches across the forehead and cluster headaches. Massaging it into the neck, shoulders, and temples (away from the eyes) can be beneficial. If stress triggers your headaches, give this calming, antispasmodic rollerball blend a try.

1 plastic pipette	2 drops balsam copaiba essential oil	10ml amber or cobalt glass rollerball bottle
3 drops frankincense essential oil		
2 drops bergamot mint essential oil	2 drops lavender essential oil	1 ounce jojoba wax

1. Using the pipette, add the essential oils to the rollerball bottle.

2. Fill the remainder of the bottle with the jojoba wax, leaving enough space at the top for the rollerball applicator so your oils do not overflow.

3. Pop in the rollerball applicator, and cap tightly.

4. Apply topically as needed.

HORMONE HELP INHALER

DIRECT INHALATION   Safe for Ages 5+

This headache blend is specifically for girls who have hit puberty and women of all ages. Hormonal fluctuations can result in PMS or menopausal symptoms, and headaches are common. Clary sage and geranium address hormonal fluctuations and, via inhalation, can stop a headache in its tracks. Alternatively, this blend of oils can be used in a diffuser or an aroma bath to relieve many hormonal symptoms and provide restorative rest.

4 plastic pipettes	5 drops clary sage essential oil	1 drop helichrysum essential oil
6 drops bergamot mint essential oil	3 drops geranium essential oil	Aromatherapy inhaler

1. Using the pipettes, place the essential oils onto the cotton wick of the inhaler, and snap the cap firmly into place.

2. Carry the inhaler with you, and open the cap and inhale slowly multiple times as needed.

JUST FOR CHILDREN

NECK AND SOLDIERS MASSAGE OIL

TOPICAL USE   Safe for Ages 2+

This blend with the fun title is formulated especially with your children in mind. Children have many moments when their muscles are overworked from sports or growth spurts. My oldest doesn't have the best posture and, as a result, has tight, knotted shoulders, but this blend helps. Rub into the desired area, and follow up with a nice, warm compress or heating pad.

4 drops lavender essential oil

2 drops Roman chamomile essential oil

2 drops sweet marjoram essential oil

1 drop geranium essential oil

1 ounce jojoba wax

1. In a glass container, blend the essential oils into the jojoba wax.

2. Use as needed to soothe your child's aches and pains, helping them rest comfortably. Store unused portion in a cool place.

SHAKE IT OFF HEADACHE TAMER ROLLERBALL BLEND

TOPICAL USE   Safe for Ages 2+

This blend is a blessing for my oldest son, who tends to get headaches with his growing pains. Lavender induces relaxation and reduces stress, which accounts for well over 50 percent of our common headaches. Roman chamomile is similar in its action and also is highly anti-inflammatory, helping address various sources of tension. Frankincense, too, addresses a variety of pains.[111]

1 plastic pipette
2 drops lavender
    essential oil
2 drops Roman
    chamomile
    essential oil

1 drop sweet
    marjoram
    essential oil
1 drop frankincense
    essential oil

10ml amber or
    cobalt glass
    rollerball bottle
~9ml carrier oil

1. Using the pipette, add the essential oils to the rollerball bottle.

2. Fill the remainder of the bottle with the carrier oil, leaving enough space at the top for the rollerball applicator so your oils do not overflow.

3. Pop in the rollerball applicator, and cap tightly.

4. Apply topically as needed.

Insomnia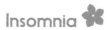

BLISSFULLY SLEEPY DIFFUSER BLEND

PASSIVE INHALATION   Safe for Ages 3+ Months

Insomnia affects many people for various reasons, and these essential oils have been shown to be effective for a restful night's sleep. This blend is sure to help you to unwind and prepare for slumber. These essential oils are not high in esters or linalool, but they support blissful rest. Start running the diffuser for 30 minutes before bedtime to prepare your room.

4 drops red mandarin essential oil

2 drops ruh khus essential oil

2 drops sandalwood essential oil

1 drop spikenard essential oil

1 drop jasmine essential oil

Place the essential oils into your favorite diffuser according to manufacturer instructions. Use this blend as needed. Follow safe diffusing guidelines.

RESTORATIVE SLEEP MASSAGE OIL

TOPICAL USE   Safe for Ages 2+

A large part of a successful sleep schedule is taking the time to wind down. Turning off electronics 30 minutes before trying to fall sleep will help ensure you can more quickly, as will using this massage blend. This synergy is rich in esters, linalool, and linalyl acetate, helping soften the body and quiet the mind. Research shows that children also benefit from a parent's or trusted caregiver's gentle touch, and the combination of that touch and these oils will help ensure a good night's sleep.[112]

5 drops lavender essential oil

2 drops ho wood essential oil

1 drop petitgrain essential oil

1 drop Roman chamomile essential oil

1 ounce grapeseed oil

1. Combine the essential oils with the grapeseed oil in a glass container.

2. Massage into the arms, chest, and legs. Use as needed. Store unused portion in a cool place.

SHUT-OFF SWITCH DIFFUSER BLEND

An astronomical 1 in 4 Americans suffers from insomnia at one time in their life, and that number is on the rise, according to a 2018 study.[113] I think one of the reasons is our inability to shut off worry and fear. Insomnia can be temporary or chronic, putting overall health at risk. Using essential oils at bedtime has helped many people find the much-needed sleep they are lacking. See if this blend works for you.

5 drops bergamot orange essential oil

2 drops frankincense essential oil

2 drops myrrh essential oil

1 drop geranium essential oil

Place the essential oils into your favorite diffuser according to manufacturer instructions. Use this blend as needed. Follow safe diffusing guidelines.

JUST FOR CHILDREN

DREAMY NIGHT DIFFUSER BLEND

PASSIVE INHALATION   Safe for Ages 3+ Months

Dreamy Night has been formulated especially for children and is safe for those ages 3 months and older if you follow the safe diffusing recommendations found in this book. According to Virginia Musacchio of Stillpoint Aromatics, Fragonia "helps regulate mental [and] emotional issues, stress, anxiety, depression, anger [and] insomnia."[114] I purchased my first bottle of Fragonia from Stillpoint Aromatics and have used it in my sleep blends ever since. This essential oil synergy will have your child sleeping in no time. Begin diffusing before they lie down for the evening.

4 drops lavender
    essential oil
3 drops Fragonia
    essential oil

2 drops red mandarin
    essential oil
1 drop spikenard
    essential oil

Place the essential oils into your favorite diffuser according to manufacturer instructions. Use this blend as needed. Follow safe diffusing guidelines.

SLEEPY EYES PILLOW SPRAY

PASSIVE INHALATION   Safe for Ages 2+

An aromatic spritzer is a great alternative to a diffuser. Under your supervision, an older child can spray it over their linens and pillow, helping them feel empowered to act if they are having issues falling asleep due to overthinking, worry, or fear. This blend smells truly divine and will help your child settle into dreamland.

7 drops sweet orange essential oil

2 drops cedarwood atlas essential oil

2 drops ylang-ylang essential oil

1 drop Roman chamomile essential oil

1 (2-ounce) glass spray bottle

½ ounce 190-proof alcohol or perfumers alcohol

Distilled water

1. Place the essential oils into the bottle.

2. Add the alcohol to help the oils dissolve.

3. Fill the remainder of the bottle with distilled water.

4. Label and store in a cool place.

SNUG AS A BUG IN A RUG DIFFUSER BLEND

PASSIVE INHALATION   Safe for Ages 3+ Months

Insomnia can strike children at any time, just like it can affect adults. Essential oils are exceptional in their ability to help promote restful sleep. Both lavender and ho wood are high in the chemical constituent linalool, a gentle but effective sedative. Roman chamomile is high in esters, helping encourage a deep sense of calm and reassurance. Frankincense is a sweet addition to the synergy because it is grounding in nature to help stop overthinking. The synergy of these four essential oils is palpable, and they smell amazing, too.

5 drops lavender essential oil

2 drops frankincense essential oil

2 drops Roman chamomile essential oil

1 drop ho wood essential oil

Place the essential oils into your favorite diffuser according to manufacturer instructions. Follow safe diffusing guidelines.

Loss of Libido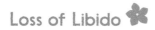

DATE NIGHT MASSAGE OIL

TOPICAL USE   Safe for Ages 2+

Although these essential oils are safe topically for children ages 2 years and older, this massage oil is for adults. A lagging libido is a very real problem, and even something as simple as stress can affect our sex drive. This massage oil helps promote relaxation and create intimacy, relieving stress and boosting our sex drive.

5 drops sweet orange essential oil	1 drops jasmine essential oil	1 ounce plain or vanilla-infused
2 drops davana essential oil	1 drop sandalwood essential oil	jojoba wax (see Tip, page 125)

1. In a glass container, blend the essential oils into the jojoba wax.

2. Set the mood and massage your partner, with no expectations other than facilitating a deep connection. Use as needed. Store unused portion in a cool place.

EMBRACING FEMININITY BATH SALTS (MASTER BLEND)

TOPICAL USE   Safe for Ages 5+

This essential oil bath recipe is for addressing the female libido. I encourage women to get in touch with their femininity as often as possible. Embrace it, cultivate it, and live it. Sexuality, femininity, and womanhood are about self, self-awareness, and expansion, and this blend encourages you to connect with the female self.

5ml dark glass bottle

20 drops sweet orange essential oil

8 drops helichrysum essential oil

7 drops rose otto essential oil

5 drops patchouli essential oil

1 tablespoon carrier oil

1 cup Epsom salts (optional)

½ cup full-fat coconut cream (optional)

1. In the glass bottle, combine the essential oils to create a master blend. Store in a cool location until ready to use.

2. Mix 5 to 7 drops of the master blend with the carrier oil, and add to the Epsom salts, if using, or directly to bathwater. If using the coconut cream, add it to the bathwater last. Quiet your mind and enjoy your soak.

LAGGING LIBIDO DIFFUSER BLEND

PASSIVE INHALATION   Safe for Ages 3+ Months

Although these essential oils are safe for diffusion for babies and children ages 3 months and older, this blend is intended for adults only. Sandalwood, one of my top five favorite essential oils, is included in this blend with men in mind. It is touted by many as having aphrodisiac properties for men, and the sultry scent of jasmine is among the most recommended essential oils to help boost a lagging libido. A little bit of this evocative scent is all that is needed. Lastly, neroli essential oil calms the nervous system to help us get in the mood.

5 drops Australian sandalwood essential oil

2 drops neroli essential oil

2 drops jasmine essential oil

1 drop ylang ylang essential oil

Place the essential oils into your favorite diffuser according to manufacturer instructions. Diffuse, and see what unfolds. Follow safe diffusing guidelines.

Falling Ill When Under Stress 🌸

CLEAN SWEEP HARD SURFACE CLEANER

PASSIVE INHALATION   Safe for Ages 2+

This essential oil blend has a relatively high recommended dilution to help sanitize hard surfaces and remove unwanted microbes from the air. Many of us want a home free of toxic chemical cleaners. Thankfully, essential oils can clean hard surfaces and kill germs, making our homes safer.

20 drops lemon essential oil

20 drops lime essential oil

12 drops cypress essential oil

10 drops Siberian fir essential oil

10 drops lavender essential oil

1 (4-ounce) glass spray bottle

1 ounce 190-proof alcohol or perfumers alcohol

Distilled water

1. Place the essential oils into the bottle.

2. Add the alcohol, and mix.

3. Fill the remainder of the bottle with distilled water. Shake.

4. Label and store in a cool place.

5. Let this spray sit on hard surfaces for 10 minutes before wiping clean.

IMMUNE SUPPORT DIFFUSER BLEND (MASTER BLEND)

If someone in the home has fallen ill, diffuse this antimicrobial blend in the home or office to help them recover faster and prevent the spread of germs. This blend is safe and effective for ages 3 months and up, unlike other, popular antigerm essential oils on the market that have potentially unsafe interactions. Give this diffuser blend a try to support your immune system.

5ml dark glass bottle

10 drops lemon essential oil

10 drops laurel leaf essential oil

10 drops sweet orange essential oil

5 drops bergamot orange essential oil

5 drops sweet marjoram essential oil

1. In the glass bottle, combine the essential oils to create a master blend. Store in a cool location until ready to use.

2. Add as desired to your favorite diffuser according to manufacturer instructions. Follow safe diffusing guidelines.

REST AND RESTORE DIFFUSER BLEND

PASSIVE INHALATION   Safe for Ages 3+ Months

Not every essential oil blend is as it seems at first glance. Even oils that are not widely considered immune enhancers do a great deal to support us. Higher levels of stress wear us down and make us more susceptible to illness, so if we lower stress levels, it makes sense that we won't get sick as often. If you know you are going through a stressful situation that may last awhile, make sure you are taking extra special care of yourself. Diffuse often, but rest even more.

4 drops lavender essential oil

3 drops sweet orange essential oil

2 drops Buddha wood essential oil

1 drop Australian sandalwood essential oil

Place the essential oils into your favorite diffuser according to manufacturer instructions. Follow safe diffusing guidelines.

JUST FOR CHILDREN

PROTECTOR DIFFUSER BLEND (MASTER BLEND)

PASSIVE INHALATION   Safe for Ages 3+ Months

If your child has fallen ill, they likely need an immune boost with emotional support. My children react very differently when they are sick; one wants comfort and solitude, whereas the other needs his mom. Diffusing this blend in our home helps them feel comfortable, safe, and supported.

5ml dark glass bottle

15 drops Siberian fir essential oil

10 drops frankincense essential oil

10 drops sweet orange essential oil

7 drops pink pepper essential oil

3 drops cedarwood atlas essential oil

1. In the glass bottle, combine the essential oils to create a master blend. Store in a cool location until ready to use.

2. Add as desired to your favorite diffuser according to manufacturer instructions. Follow safe diffusing guidelines.

Post-traumatic Stress Disorder (PTSD)/Trauma

BREAK THE CYCLE DIFFUSER BLEND

PASSIVE INHALATION   Safe for Ages 3+ Months

Individuals dealing with trauma and PTSD need support, and that may look different from one individual to the next. Shock, trauma, and the parasympathetic system go hand in hand. These essential oils support the body while encouraging the mind to stay steady, the heart to soften and open, and the nervous system to remain strong. To those who are suffering, know that you are not alone. Please ask for help.

4 drops cistus
    essential oil
3 drops helichrysum
    essential oil

2 drops frankincense
    essential oil
1 drop rose otto
    essential oil

Place the essential oils into your favorite diffuser according to manufacturer instructions. Follow safe diffusing guidelines.

GAIN PERSPECTIVE AROMATHERAPY INHALER

DIRECT INHALATION   Safe for Ages 5+

For individuals dealing with trauma and PTSD, having a portable aromatherapy inhaler can be important, since a trigger might present itself at any time. If your trauma has you feeling anger that needs release, yarrow essential oil can help you express yourself in a healthier, more positive way. Helichrysum also helps give you the courage to know you can handle anything that life throws at you.

4 plastic pipettes	4 drops bergamot orange essential oil	2 drops helichrysum essential oil
5 drops yarrow essential oil	4 drops lime essential oil	Aromatherapy inhaler

1. Using the pipettes, place the essential oils onto the cotton wick of the inhaler, and snap the cap firmly into place.

2. Carry the inhaler with you, and open the cap and inhale slowly multiple times to alleviate anxiety when it strikes.

REST AND DIGEST ANOINTING OIL

TOPICAL USE   Safe for Ages 2+

Most individuals with PTSD manifest emotions in several ways, including nightmares, panic attacks, and an overall, constant sense of anxiety. Whether this description applies to you or someone you love, seeking therapy is incredibly important for you to live a long, happy life. I recommend this anointing oil for a sense of protection before you leave the house for the day or before bedtime so you can benefit from the therapeutics while you sleep.

4 drops lavender essential oil

2 drops clary sage essential oil

2 drops angelica root essential oil

1 drop geranium essential oil

1 ounce jojoba wax

1. In a glass container, blend the essential oils into the jojoba wax.

2. Apply as needed, anointing your chakras and inhaling deeply. Store the unused portion in a cool place.

Seasonal Affective Disorder (SAD)

PASSIVE INHALATION   Safe for Ages 3+ Months

SAD is a common mood disorder in the northern hemisphere.[115] The further north you live, the less sun you get in the wintertime. Help comes in the form of light therapy, an additional intake of vitamin D, and essential oils, to name a few treatments. By far, citrus oils are the most researched essential oils for depression and altered mood states.[116] Direct inhalation of a combination of citrus oils can improve mood and greatly help those suffering from SAD, and this blend is the first of three I suggest.

4 drops lemon   2 drops bergamot   1 drop jasmine
    essential oil   orange   essential oil
3 drops red mandarin   essential oil
    essential oil

Place the essential oils into your favorite diffuser according to manufacturer instructions. Follow safe diffusing guidelines.

WINTER'S SLUMBER DIFFUSER BLEND

PASSIVE INHALATION   Safe for Ages 3+ Months

Bright-light therapy in combination with essential oil inhalation is more effective in the treatment of SAD than either treatment alone, according to one 2016 study.[117] The results of the study showed reduced blood pressure, lower heart rate, and overall improved mood. Try this blend in your diffuser while you are getting ready to start the day. It can benefit the entire family.

4 drops bergamot orange essential oil

3 drops pink pepper essential oil

2 drops lavender essential oil

1 drop petitgrain essential oil

Place the essential oils into your favorite diffuser according to manufacturer instructions. Follow safe diffusing guidelines.

WISHING FOR SPRING AROMATHERAPY INHALER

DIRECT INHALATION   Safe for Ages 5+

Roman chamomile is very calming and has been found to be possibly useful for the treatment of generalized anxiety disorder, which is often a result of SAD, one study showed.[118] Its effects are mild to moderate, but when it is used in synergy with citrus essential oils, you can feel a palpable difference. Keep this portable aromatherapy inhaler with you throughout the day when your mood needs a boost.

5 plastic pipettes

6 drops sweet orange essential oil

3 drops red mandarin essential oil

3 drops marjoram essential oil

2 drops Roman chamomile essential oil

1 drop vetiver essential oil

Aromatherapy inhaler

1. Using the pipettes, place the essential oils onto the cotton wick of the inhaler, and snap the cap firmly into place.

2. Carry the inhaler with you, and open the cap and inhale slowly multiple times in gloomy winter months as needed.

Meditation/Yoga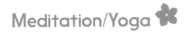

BREATHE IN, BREATHE OUT DIFFUSER BLEND

PASSIVE INHALATION   Safe for Ages 3+ Months

Breathe In, Breathe Out Diffuser Blend can restore calm in turbulent moments. Cape chamomile will bring you back in balance and breathing fully again. Buddha wood, when combined with cape chamomile, helps ground you to Mother Earth when you feel airy and anxious. Lastly, lavender, with a little addition of blue tansy, is protective and uplifting. Try this blend when you feel panic coming on, or use it in advance before an event that you know will upset or agitate you.

4 drops cape chamomile essential oil

3 drops lavender essential oil

2 drops Buddha wood essential oil

1 drop blue tansy essential oil

Place the essential oils into your favorite diffuser according to manufacturer instructions. Follow safe diffusing guidelines.

FIND YOUR ZEN DIFFUSER BLEND (MASTER BLEND)

PASSIVE INHALATION   Safe for Ages 3+ Months

Elemi essential oil is highlighted in this blend for its lemony, spicy, warm aroma and its ability to help you feel safe and at one with yourself and your surroundings. Cardamom and sweet orange round out this delicious synergy of oils to use during any of your favorite self-care rituals, such as journaling, yoga, meditation, or soaking in the tub.

5ml glass bottle

10 drops cardamom essential oil

10 drops sweet orange essential oil

10 drops elemi essential oil

5 drops ruh khus essential oil

5 drops Australian sandalwood essential oil

1. In the glass bottle, combine the essential oils to create a master blend. Store in a cool location until ready to use.

2. Add as desired to your favorite diffuser according to manufacturer instructions. Follow safe diffusing guidelines.

SPIRITUAL AWAKENING DIFFUSER BLEND

Do you feel like you are on the edge of a breakthrough? Have you been working diligently on self-improvement and feel like you are standing on the brink of a revelation or spiritual awakening? Go with those feelings, and believe they can be true for you. This diffuser blend can help support you during this time to stand in your truth and realize your power. This synergy is extremely uplifting and supportive, giving you the vibes you need to realize this is the time to take action in your life.

4 drops bergamot orange essential oil

3 drops cistus essential oil

2 drops myrrh essential oil

1 drop neroli essential oil

Place the essential oils into your favorite diffuser according to the manufacturer instructions. Follow safe diffusing guidelines.

Protective Blends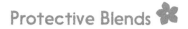

PASSIVE INHALATION   Safe for Ages 5+

This uplifting, energizing, yet grounding aromatherapy inhaler blend is perfect when you are feeling misunderstood, antsy, and irritable. The tree essential oils in this blend are supportive of our growth while maintaining our roots. Reach for this synergy to help guide you toward a clear expression of your thoughts and feelings when kind and compassionate communication is needed. Speak your truth, strengthen your resolve, and take that next step toward healing.

4 plastic pipettes	3 drops cypress essential oil	1 drop Siberian fir essential oil
8 drops lime essential oil	3 drops black spruce essential oil	Aromatherapy inhaler

1. Using the pipettes, place the essential oils onto the cotton wick of the inhaler, and snap the cap firmly into place.

2. Carry the inhaler with you, and open the cap and inhale slowly multiple times as needed.

PERSONAL SANCTUARY PERFUME

This unique blend of oils in a base of jojoba wax lets you bring your personal sanctuary with you wherever you go. Cedarwood atlas is the highlight of the perfume, with its ability to conjure endurance, strength, and resilience. Remember how powerful you are with this stunning essential oil. Jasmine and ylang-ylang smooth the edges of cedarwood atlas and vetiver, adding divine heady and floral aromas.

4 drops cedarwood atlas essential oil

2 drops jasmine essential oil

2 drop vetiver essential oil

1 drop ylang-ylang essential oil

9 drops plain or vanilla-infused jojoba wax (see Tip, page 125)

1. In a glass container, blend the essential oils into the jojoba wax.

2. Apply to points on neck and wrists, massaging into your skin. Store unused portion in a cool place.

PURE ENERGY DIFFUSER BLEND

TOPICAL USE   Safe for Ages 3+ Months

Although these essential oils are safe aromatically for children ages 3 months and older, this energetic blend is geared toward older children and adults who feel anxious. Frankincense is perhaps one of the most energy-protective essential oils in existence. Its aroma is sweet and light. Palo santo guards our emotional space when we are overwhelmed with the negative energies of others, and rose helps protect us while keep our hearts open and strong.

5 drops frankincense   2 drops palo santo
    essential oil   essential oil
2 drops myrrh   1 drop rose otto
    essential oil   essential oil

Place the essential oils into your favorite diffuser according to manufacturer instructions. Follow safe diffusing guidelines. Alternatively, you can adjust the number of drops for an aromatherapy inhaler to be used in crowded or loud public spaces.

Self-Care Sanctuary ❀

AROMATHERAPY BATHS

TOPICAL USE   Safe for Ages 5+

Self-care is incredibly important, and it should be a daily habit. The more bliss we can welcome into our life, the more our mind and body will be deliciously calm and at ease. Cardamom is indicated for worry and to help bring balance and clarity. Rose is all about the heart, softening, opening, trusting, and self-love. Warning: You may never want to get out of the bathtub, so lock the door.

4 drops cardamom essential oil	1 tablespoon carrier oil	½ cup full-fat coconut cream (optional)
3 drops rose otto essential oil	1 cup Epsom salts (optional)	

In a glass container, mix the essential oils with the carrier oil, and add to the Epsom salts, if using, or directly to the bathwater. If using the coconut cream, add it to the bath last.

PAMPERED AND PEACEFUL BATH BALL

TOPICAL USE   Safe for Ages 5+

Pamper yourself with this heavenly, floral blend of essential oils to prepare for a night of deep sleep.

1 cup baking soda
½ cup citric acid
½ cup arrowroot
    powder
2 ¼ tablespoons
    grapeseed oil
½ tablespoon
    vanilla extract

20 drops lavender
    essential oil
10 drops geranium
    essential oil
8 drops petitgrain
    essential oil
2 drops jasmine
    essential oil

¾ tablespoon
    distilled water
Your favorite
    stainless steel or
    silicone molds

1. Mix the baking soda, citric acid, and arrowroot powder in a bowl.

2. In a separate bowl, blend the grapeseed oil, vanilla extract, essential oils, and water.

3. Slowly combine the wet and dry ingredients, blending until mixed well.

4. Use molds to form into balls.

5. Let sit to dry and harden.

6. Use one ball at a time once you are in the bath, dropping it into the water.

PARADISE FIZZY BATH BALL

Close your eyes and picture yourself on a sunny beach.
Don't forget your umbrella drink.

1 cup baking soda
½ cup citric acid
½ cup arrowroot
    powder
2 ¼ tablespoons
    grapeseed oil
½ tablespoon
    vanilla extract

¾ tablespoon
    distilled water
20 drops sweet
    orange
    essential oil
7 drops red mandarin
    essential oil
5 drops cardamom
    essential oil

5 drops Australian
    sandalwood
    essential oil
3 drops ylang-ylang
    essential oil
Your favorite
    stainless steel or
    silicone molds

1. Mix the baking soda, citric acid, and arrowroot powder in a bowl.

2. Blend the grapeseed oil, vanilla extract, water, and essential oils in a separate bowl.

3. Slowly combine the wet and dry ingredients, blending consistently until mixed well.

4. Use molds to form into balls.

5. Let sit to dry and harden.

6. Use one ball at a time once you are in the bath, dropping it into the water.

BREAST OIL

BREAST HEALTH SYNERGY

TOPICAL USE   Safe for Ages 2+, Phototoxic

This blend is intended for women as part of a breast self-care routine. Massage daily into your breast tissue, including the upper-right quadrant near the armpit. Massage in slow circles and give yourself some quality self-love. This is a great preventive routine that I've adapted from Robert Tisserand's online recipe.[119]

10 drops lemon
   essential oil
5 drops bergamot
   orange
   essential oil

5 drops pink pepper
   essential oil
6 drops balsam
   copaiba
   essential oil

3 drops cedarwood
   atlas essential oil
2 ounces pomegranate
   carrier oil
2 ounces rosehip seed
   carrier oil

Blend the essential oils with the pomegranate and rosehip seed oils in a glass container for daily use. Store unused portion in a cool location. If applying immediately after bathing, be sure not to introduce any moisture into the container, which would encourage microbial growth.

FOOT SOAKS

INVIGORATING FOOT SOAK

TOPICAL USE   Safe for Ages 5+

Try this invigorating foot soak for tired feet. It's a great self-care exercise after a long day, and it's especially useful before giving yourself a pedicure.

2 drops bergamot mint essential oil

2 drops sweet orange essential oil

1 tablespoon jojoba wax

½ cup Epsom salts

¼ cup pink Himalayan sea salt

Mix the essential oils, jojoba wax, Epsom salts, and Himalayan sea salt well in a glass or stainless steel bowl of warm water. Enjoy a soak for your tired, aching feet.

WARMING FOOT SOAK

TOPICAL USE   Safe for Ages 5+

This warming blend of cardamom, red mandarin, and rose is a welcome respite after a busy day. Grab your favorite book and indulge a little. You deserve it.

2 drops cardamom essential oil

1 drop red mandarin essential oil

1 drop rose otto essential oil

1 tablespoon jojoba wax

½ cup Epsom salts

¼ cup pink Himalayan sea salt

Mix the essential oils, jojoba wax, Epsom salts, and Himalayan sea salt well in a glass or stainless steel bowl of warm water. Enjoy a soak for your tired, aching feet.

SCRUBS

TOPICAL USE   For Adults

This sugar scrub is best for adults to help exfoliate and pamper the skin. It should not be used with children, who have more sensitive skin.

10 drops Australian
    sandalwood
    essential oil
5 drops lavender
    essential oil

5 drops clary sage
    essential oil
½ cup coconut oil
    or extra-virgin
    olive oil

1 cup granulated
    sugar,
    preferably
    organic

1. In a small glass jar with a lid, mix the essential oils, coconut oil, and sugar.

2. Use the scrub in the shower or tub before you run the water, then rinse off. Make sure not to dip wet fingers into the container, to avoid contaminating unused scrub.

ENERGIZING COFFEE SCRUB

TOPICAL USE   For Adults

I use a coffee scrub once or twice a week. As a result, I rarely need to moisturize my skin throughout the week. After having my morning coffee (one serving), I place the wet grounds in a small bowl and use them to make this scrub.

~2 tablespoons wet coffee grounds

1 tablespoon extra-virgin olive oil

1 teaspoon organic vanilla extract OR

3 drops essential oil (such as Roman chamomile, frankincense, lavender, or bergamot mint)

1. In a small glass jar with a lid, mix the coffee grounds, olive oil, and vanilla extract or essential oil.

2. Use the scrub in the shower or tub before you run the water, then rinse off. Make sure not to dip wet fingers into the container to avoid contaminating unused scrub.

ULTIMATE EXFOLIATOR

Do you have calloused hands from gardening in the dirt or flaking heels from walking barefoot too often? This blend is my ultimate exfoliator recipe, meant only for the rougher skin areas, like the hands, feet, and elbows.

10 drops cedarwood atlas essential oil

7 drops balsam copaiba essential oil

½ cup extra-virgin olive oil

2 tablespoons raw honey, softened

2 cups granulated sugar, preferably organic

1. In a glass container, mix the essential oils with the olive oil, and add the honey and sugar. Mix well.

2. Massage in a circular motion into rough areas, and rinse.

CHAKRA BALANCING SET

ROOT CHAKRA: FIND YOUR ROOTS ROLLERBALL BLEND

TOPICAL USE   For Adults

Our root chakra represents stability, which includes our basic survival needs, such as shelter, food, and water, and feeling at home in our body and on this planet.[120] Grounding yourself is the most important practice for your root chakra to feel safe and protected. Use this blend to help.

1 plastic pipette	3 drops frankincense essential oil	10ml amber or cobalt glass rollerball bottle
5 drops grapefruit essential oil	2 drops vetiver essential oil	~9ml carrier oil

1. Using the pipette, add the essential oils to the rollerball bottle.

2. Fill the remainder of the bottle with the carrier oil, leaving enough space at the top for the rollerball applicator so your oils do not overflow.

3. Pop in the rollerball applicator, and cap tightly.

4. Apply topically as needed.

SACRAL CHAKRA: EMBODY YOUR MUSE ROLLERBALL BLEND

TOPICAL USE   For Adults

Our sacral chakra represents our creativity, our sensuality, and all of our senses.[121] To find balance in this chakra, we need to focus on the flow and fluidity of our creative side, to practice things that bring us pleasure, and to use our senses regularly with deep intention.

1 plastic pipette
5 drops orange essential oil

3 drops Australian sandalwood essential oil
2 drops rose otto essential oil

10ml amber or cobalt glass rollerball bottle
~9ml carrier oil

1. Using the pipette, add the essential oils to the rollerball bottle.

2. Fill the remainder of the bottle with the carrier oil, leaving enough space at the top for the rollerball applicator so your oils do not overflow.

3. Pop in the rollerball applicator, and cap tightly.

4. Apply topically as needed.

SOLAR PLEXUS CHAKRA: MANIFEST POTENTIAL ROLLERBALL BLEND

TOPICAL USE   For Adults

Our solar plexus chakra represents our personal power, our identity, and taking back control of our life.[122] To find balance in this chakra, we need to get in touch with our feelings, behaviors, and emotions, as I discussed at the beginning of the book. These oils work to assist in this process.

1 plastic pipette	3 drops davana essential oil	10ml amber or cobalt glass rollerball bottle
5 drops cardamom essential oil	2 drops black pepper essential oil	~9ml carrier oil

1. Using the pipette, add the essential oils to the rollerball bottle.

2. Fill the remainder of the bottle with the carrier oil, leaving enough space at the top for the rollerball applicator so your oils do not overflow.

3. Pop in the rollerball applicator, and cap tightly.

4. Apply topically as needed.

HEART CHAKRA: UNCONDITIONAL LOVE ROLLERBALL BLEND

TOPICAL USE   For Adults

Our heart chakra is all about love—love for others and ourselves.[123] Have you ever had your heart broken? Felt the deep sense of loss of a loved one? Your heart chakra was affected. Nurturing forgiveness and self-compassion are important during this chapter of your life.

1 plastic pipette	3 drops balsam copaiba essential oil	10ml amber or cobalt glass rollerball bottle
5 drops lime essential oil	2 drops rhododendron essential oil	~9ml carrier oil

1. Using the pipette, add the essential oils to the rollerball bottle.

2. Fill the remainder of the bottle with the carrier oil, leaving enough space at the top for the rollerball applicator so your oils do not overflow.

3. Pop in the rollerball applicator, and cap tightly.

4. Apply topically as needed.

THROAT CHAKRA: CLEAR EXPRESSION ROLLERBALL BLEND

TOPICAL USE   For Adults

Clear expression, speaking our truth, having healthy boundaries—all of these things are represented by the throat chakra.[124] This chakra supports seeing what is true for us and not allowing our ego to make up stories, or what I sometimes have referred to as our "inner mean girl/boy." Use this blend to help support your clear expression.

1 plastic pipette
5 drops clary sage
   essential oil
3 drops blue tansy
   essential oil

2 drops Roman
   chamomile
   essential oil

10ml amber or
   cobalt glass
   rollerball bottle
~9ml carrier oil

1. Using the pipette, add the essential oils to the rollerball bottle.

2. Fill the remainder of the bottle with the carrier oil, leaving enough space at the top for the rollerball applicator so your oils do not overflow.

3. Pop in the rollerball applicator, and cap tightly.

4. Apply topically as needed.

THIRD EYE CHAKRA: PEACEFUL AWARENESS ROLLERBALL BLEND

TOPICAL USE   For Adults

Our third eye represents our inner being or our intuition. This area is said to be where we transcend duality, or the physical separation of self from the rest of the world.[125] Here, we are the world, and the world is in us. Apply this oil to the third eye during meditation.

1 plastic pipette

5 drops red mandarin essential oil

3 drops patchouli essential oil

2 drops elemi essential oil

10ml amber or cobalt glass rollerball bottle

~9ml carrier oil

1. Using the pipette, add the essential oils to the rollerball bottle.

2. Fill the remainder of the bottle with the carrier oil, leaving enough space at the top for the rollerball applicator so your oils do not overflow.

3. Pop in the rollerball applicator, and cap tightly.

4. Apply topically as needed.

CROWN CHAKRA: HIGHER SOURCE ROLLERBALL BLEND

TOPICAL USE   For Adults

The crown chakra, located at the top of the head, is our deep connection to Mother Earth. When this chakra is in balance, you have a clear connection to your belief system, your higher states of consciousness, and in terms of emotional wellness, your ability to release any limiting beliefs you have about yourself.[126]

1 plastic pipette	3 drops neroli essential oil	10ml amber or cobalt glass rollerball bottle
5 drops lavender essential oil	2 drops jasmine essential oil	~9ml carrier oil

1. Using the pipette, add the essential oils to the rollerball bottle.

2. Fill the remainder of the bottle with the carrier oil, leaving enough space at the top for the rollerball applicator so your oils do not overflow.

3. Pop in the rollerball applicator, and cap tightly.

4. Apply topically as needed.

Resources

Books

Murray, Michael T., and Joseph E. Pizzorno. *The Encyclopedia of Natural Medicine.* 3rd ed. New York: Atria Books, 2012.

> This best seller is the most important resource in my toolbox for alternative and complementary medicine. Covering more than 80 ailments, including many for emotional wellness, this book is a must-have.

Parker, Susan. *Power of the Seed: Your Guide to Oils for Health and Beauty.* Port Townsend, WA: Process Media, 2015.

> This very thorough book on carrier oils is an additional resource for you to learn more about quality carrier oils for your aromatherapy blending.

Price, Shirley, and Len Price. *Aromatherapy for Health Professionals.* 4th ed. London: Churchill Livingstone, 2011.

> This book has been a valued reference volume on my bookshelf for several years. Look for it if you want comprehensive, clinical-based aromatherapy information.

Rhind, Jennifer Peace. *Aromatherapeutic Blending: Essential Oils in Synergy.* London and Philadelphia: Singing Dragon, 2015.

> *Aromatherapeutic Blending* goes into great detail about the synergy of essential oils and how you can harness it in your own blending at home. Many essential oils are profiled, along with research studies. Resources also are provided for further reading.

Websites

Active Meditation. "Mini Meditations: Accessible Exercises for Everyday Use." www.activemeditation.org/mini-meditations.

AromaWeb. "Essential Oils and Aromatherapy Resources." www.aromaweb.com.

Gaiam. "Meditation 101: Techniques, Benefits, and a Beginner's How-to." www.gaiam.com/blogs/discover/meditation-101-techniques-benefits-and-a-beginner-s-how-to.

Mindful. "Healthy Mind, Healthy Life." www.mindful.org.

Tapping Solution Foundation. "Promoting the Healing Effects of EFT Tapping to People of All Ages around the World." www.tappingsolutionfoundation.org.

Tisserand Institute. "The Complete Skin Series by Robert Tisserand." tisserandinstitute.org/online-courses/complete-skin-series/.

Essential Oil Sources

Aromatics International. www.aromatics.com.

Eden Botanicals. www.edenbotanicals.com.

Stillpoint Aromatics. www.stillpointaromatics.com.

Emotions Chart

EMOTION	PHYSICAL SYMPTOMS	EMOTIONAL DESCRIPTORS	RECOMMENDATION
Anger	Increased blood pressure, headache, heart palpitations, paranoia, social isolation	Anxious, disgusted, furious, irrational, irritated, livid, resentful	Release the Anger Aromatherapy Inhaler (page 109)
Anxiety	Chest tightness, dry mouth, shakiness, limb numbness, racing heartbeat, shortness of breath	Fidgety, catastrophic-type thinking, distressed, feeling of out of control, jittery, panicked, restless	Kiss Overwhelm Goodbye Aromatherapy Inhaler (page 102)
Depression	Excessive crying, fatigue, headache, insomnia, isolation, pain, constant sleeping, withdrawal	Angry, feeling desolation and despair, forlorn, hopeless, hurting, pessimistic, sad, tearful, unhappy	The Sun Will Come Out Diffuser Blend (page 111)
Detachment	Brain fog, out-of-body feeling, isolation, poor concentration, panic attacks, tingling extremities	Alienated, anxious, depersonalized, empty, isolated, lost, numb, unmotivated, withdrawn, worried	Pure Energy Diffuser Blend (page 178)

EMOTION	PHYSICAL SYMPTOMS	EMOTIONAL DESCRIPTORS	RECOMMENDATION
Exhaustion	Changes in appetite, digestive problems, weight loss or gain	Anxious, irritable, overworked, pessimistic	Silver Lining Diffuser Blend (page 170)
Fatigue	Forgetfulness, sleepless nights, fatigue, heavy limbs	Feeling detached, helpless, irritable, short-tempered, weepy	Refreshed and Alert Aromatherapy Inhaler (page 120)
Fear	Nausea, rapid heartbeat, sweating, trembling	Anxious, embarrassed, having irrational thoughts, nervous, stressed, worried	Clear the Energy Room Spray (page 116)
Frustration	Fidgeting, jaw clenching, chest tightness, crying, sighing	Aggravated, angry, annoyed, defeated, disappointed	Slow Down Frown Diffuser Blend (page 104)
Gloominess/ Seasonal affective disorder	Aches and pains, appetite changes, heavy limbs, oversleeping	Anxious, apathetic, irritable, isolated, unmotivated, tired, moody	Winter's Slumber Diffuser Blend (page 171)
Grief	Headache, pain, heartaches, insomnia, lack of appetite	Angry, in denial, feeling despair, miserable, sad, upset	Soften the Heart Body Oil (page 110)

EMOTION	PHYSICAL SYMPTOMS	EMOTIONAL DESCRIPTORS	RECOMMENDATION
Hopelessness/ Post-traumatic stress disorder	Depression, decrease in concentration, flashbacks, memory issues, nightmares, pain	Alienated, avoidant, guilty, feeling helpless, hyperaroused, numb, overwhelmed, self-blaming	Rest and Digest Anointing Oil (page 169)
Irritability	Hot flashes, increased heart rate, rapid breathing, reduced sex drive	Angry, annoyed, confused, impatient, moody, testy, resentful	Bright and Cheerful Diffuser Blend (page 115)
Lethargy	Depression, weakness, heavy limbs, lowered immune system, slowed reflexes	Apathetic, feeling dull or in a stupor, exhausted, numb, unmotivated, weary	Spiritual Awakening Diffuser Blend (page 175)
Loss	Headaches, aches and pains, insomnia, physical tightness in the chest, shortness of breath	Angry, confused, in denial, feeling disbelief, grieving, numb, sad, in shock	Break the Cycle Diffuser Blend (page 167)
Low self-esteem	Behavioral inhibition, depression, hyperalertness to surroundings, paranoia, trauma	Critical, fearful of making mistakes, fragile, inadequate, judgmental, lacking confidence, negative	Oh, Happy Day Shower Melt (page 103)

EMOTION	PHYSICAL SYMPTOMS	EMOTIONAL DESCRIPTORS	RECOMMENDATION
Melancholy	Changes in appetite, fatigue, insomnia, weight gain	Gloomy, somber, despondent, heavy-hearted	Find Your Enthusiasm Diffuser Blend (page 117)
Mental fatigue	Chronic fatigue, decline in productivity, headaches, insomnia, loss of appetite, memory issues, mental fog	Angry, apathetic, detached, feeling dread, isolated, pessimistic, sensitive, unmotivated	Rejuvenation Diffuser Blend (page 131)
Moodiness	Chronic fatigue, difficulty concentrating, short temper	Angry, annoyed, apathetic, impatient, irritable, moody, testy, resentful	Restore Tranquility Aromatherapy Inhaler (page 130)
Negativity	Irritability, increased risk of heart disease, sleep disorders, increased stress	Hostile, uncertain, low self-esteem, pessimistic, self-pity	Bright and Blissful Anointing Oil (page 105)
Nervousness	Headache, low energy, rapid heart rate, upset stomach	Anxious, apprehensive, edgy, fearful, high-strung, jumpy, worried	Inspiring Hope Bath Salts (page 108)

EMOTION	PHYSICAL SYMPTOMS	EMOTIONAL DESCRIPTORS	RECOMMENDATION
Overthinking	Endocrine challenges, mental exhaustion	Anxious, catastrophizing, irritable, low self-esteem, nervous, overanalyzing, critical, uneasy	Stop Overthinking Aromatherapy Inhaler (page 101)
Feeling overwhelmed	Exhaustion, lightheadedness, nausea, rapid heartbeat, trouble breathing	Dazed, exhausted, overloaded, pressured, smothered	Peaceful Aura Body Oil (page 99)
Pain	Headaches, limited mobility, limited activity, stomach issues	Angry, anxious, ashamed, depressed, embarrassed, feeling misunderstood, stressed	Muscle Calm Massage Oil (page 134)
Panic	Chest pains, lightheadedness, nausea, rapid heartbeat, sweating, tingling extremities, trouble breathing	Absentminded, confused, detached, feeling dread, hysterical, intensely fearful, tense, unable to focus, unsteady	Rest and Digest Anointing Oil (page 169)
Powerlessness	Irritability, sleep disorders, inability to concentrate, increased stress	Restless, unproductive, useless, vulnerable, worthless	Grounding Rollerball Blend (page 146)

EMOTION	PHYSICAL SYMPTOMS	EMOTIONAL DESCRIPTORS	RECOMMENDATION
Self-doubt	Headaches, insomnia, increased stress, isolation, pain, pessimism	Anxious, depressed, irritable, low self-esteem, nervous, overanalyzing, perfectionism, uneasy	Have Faith Diffuser Blend (page 98)
Stress	Aches and pains, clenched jaw, chest pain, dizziness, frequent colds and illness, insomnia, low energy, rapid heartbeat, upset stomach	Agitated, defensive, depressed, frazzled, isolated, lonely, moody, negative, overwhelmed, anxious	Stress Ache Body Oil (page 136)
Feeling stuck	Irritability, sleep disorders, inability to concentrate, increased stress	Confused, detached, empty, uncertain, unmotivated, useless, vulnerable	Rest Easy Bath Salts (page 129)
Tension	Headaches, pain, knotted shoulders, low energy, poor posture, stomach upset	Anxious, depressed, irritable, overwhelmed	Pressure Release Massage Oil (page 149)
Trauma/ Post-traumatic stress disorder	Decrease in concentration, flashbacks, memory issues, nightmares, pain	Angry, anxious, avoidant, depressed, fearful, feeling out of control, irritable, ashamed	Gain Perspective Aromatherapy Inhaler (page 168)

EMOTION	PHYSICAL SYMPTOMS	EMOTIONAL DESCRIPTORS	RECOMMENDATION
Lack of focus	Exhaustion, fatigue, foggy brain, low energy	Angry, anxious, frustrated, impulsive, lost, numb, uneasy	Root Chakra: Find Your Roots Rollerball Blend (page 188)
Feeling withdrawn	Depression, fatigue, headaches, insomnia, isolation, pain, pessimism	Feeling desolate, despairing, forlorn, hopeless, hurting, lost, numb, pessimistic, vulnerable	Finding Solace Diffuser Blend (page 107)
Worry	Dizziness, irregular heartbeat, inability to concentrate, insomnia, trembling/twitching	Anxious, irritable, low self-esteem, nervous, overly concerned with what others think, critical, uneasy	Shut-Off Switch Diffuser Blend (page 156)

Essential Oils Chart

ESSENTIAL OIL	USED TO TREAT	DESIRED OUTCOME
Angelica Root	Chronic overthinking, negativity, worry	Calm, cheerful, optimistic
Balsam Copaiba	Anxiety, depression, trauma	Calm, tranquil
Basil, Sweet	Mental fog and fatigue, lack of motivation	Energized, focused, uplifted
Bergamot Orange	Depression, insomnia, fatigue	Balanced, relaxed, uplifted
Bergamot Mint	Gloominess, stress, tension	Clear, harmonious, happy
Black Pepper	Absent-mindedness, fatigue, fear	Alert, energized, focused
Black Spruce	Exhaustion, feeling overwhelmed	Calm, revitalized, stimulated
Blue Tansy	Angst, overthinking, impatience	Flexible, focused, relaxed

ESSENTIAL OIL	USED TO TREAT	DESIRED OUTCOME
Buddha Wood	Detachment, feeling frazzled or jittery	Grounded, contemplative, mindful
Cardamom	Panic, sadness, worry	Nurtured, calm, soothed
Cedarwood Atlas	Insecurity, weakness, being withdrawn	Resilient, strong
Chamomile, Cape	Apprehension, jumpiness, feeling overwhelmed	Mindful, placid, tranquil
Chamomile, Roman	Irritability, nervous tension, panic	Settled, nourished, calm
Cistus	Hysteria, shock, trauma,	Comforted, protected, settled
Clary Sage	Exhaustion, melancholy, jitters	Balanced, mildly euphoric, rested
Cypress	Feeling frazzled, nervousness, numbness	Balanced, stable, strong
Davana	Loneliness, moodiness, uncertainty	Brightened, elevated, spirited
Elemi	Apprehension, fear, withdrawal	Compassionate, content, calm
Fragonia	Imbalance, lack of motivation, feeling stuck	Harmonious, balanced, encouraged

ESSENTIAL OIL	USED TO TREAT	DESIRED OUTCOME
Frankincense	Fear, distress, weakness	Cleansed, introspective, protected
Galbanum	Agitation, distress	Assured, calm, strong
Geranium	Moodiness, PMS, restlessness	Balanced, revitalized, uplifted
Grapefruit	Depression, lethargy, sadness	Cheerful, content, lighthearted
Helichrysum	Grief, hopelessness, loss	Compassionate, encouraged, forgiving
Hemp	Distress, feeling overloaded	Reassured, relieved, softened
Ho Wood	Feelings of dread, nervousness, stress	Free, serene, still
Jasmine	Anguish, despondence, frustration	Hopeful, peaceful, comforted
Laurel Leaf	Low self-esteem, negativity, self-doubt	Confident, positive
Lavandin	Pain, restlessness, tension	Calm, pain-free, supported
Lavender	Distress, exhaustion, stress	Content, self-assured, softened

ESSENTIAL OIL	USED TO TREAT	DESIRED OUTCOME
Lemon	Agitation, anguish, sadness	Energized, optimistic, revitalized
Lime	Exhaustion, overthinking, lack of focus	Refreshed, vibrant, focused
Mandarin, Red	Confusion, lack of motivation	Compassionate, content, reawakened
Marjoram, Sweet	Grief, loss, obsessive thinking	Comforted, nurtured, rational
Myrrh	Numbness, lack of motivation, imbalance	Harmonious, peaceful, stabilized
Neroli	Feelings of distance, uncertainty, withdrawal	Clear, settled, undisturbed
Orange, Sweet	Anxiety, worry, feelings of unworthiness	Faithful, harmonious, joyful
Palo Santo	Detachment, pessimism, imbalance	Connected, dynamic, clear-sighted
Patchouli	Feelings of distance, emptiness, melancholy	Free, serene, unconditionally loved
Petitgrain	Lack of focus, overthinking, worry	Clear-sighted, peaceful, relieved
Pink Pepper	Angst, gloominess, nervousness	Encouraged, expansive, upbeat

ESSENTIAL OIL	USED TO TREAT	DESIRED OUTCOME
Rhododendron	Isolation, negativity, vulnerability	Brave, confident, open
Rose Otto	Depression, grief, loss	Forgiving, healed, open-hearted
Ruh Khus	Anger, fatigue, irritability	Balanced, grounded, satisfied
Sandalwood	Pressure, overthinking, self-criticism	Peaceful, quiet, unified
Siberian Fir	Overanalyzing, uneasiness, feeling ungrounded	Steady, strong, confident
Spikenard	Exhaustion, frayed nerves, upset	Rested, restored, self-compassionate
Vetiver	Feeling high-strung, hyperactivity, imbalance	Reassured, self-confident, stable
Yarrow	Anger, trauma	Graceful, good-natured, understanding
Ylang-Ylang	Fear, mood swings, nervous tension	Clear, harmonious, unafraid

General Index

M

O

P

Application and Remedy Index

Conditions Index

Endnotes

1   Leah Morgan, "History of Essential Oils," Healingscents, accessed June 5, 2019, https://healing scents.net/blogs/learn/18685859-history-of-essential-oils.

2   Dalinda Isabel Sánchez-Vidaña, Shirley Pui-Ching Ngai, Wanjia He, Jason Ka-Wing Chow, Benson Wui-Man Lau, and Hector Wing-Hong Tsang, "The Effectiveness of Aromatherapy for Depressive Symptoms: A Systematic Review," *Evidence-Based Complementary and Alternative Medicine* (January 2017): 1–21, doi:10.1155/2017/5869315.

3   Babar Ali, Naser Ali Al-Wabel, Saiba Shams, Aftab Ahamad, Shah Alam Khan, and Firoz Anwar, "Essential Oils Used in Aromatherapy: A Systemic Review," *Asian Pacific Journal of Tropical Biomedicine* 5, no. 8 (2015): 601–11, doi:10.1016/j.apjtb.2015.05.007.

4   Thich Nhất Hạnh, *Peace Is Every Step: The Path of Mindfulness in Everyday Life* (New York: Bantam/AJP, 1992).

5   Jane Buckle, *Clinical Aromatherapy: Essential Oils in Healthcare* (St. Louis: Elsevier, 2015), 286–301.

6   Marieke B. Toffolo, Monique A.M. Smeets, and Marcel A. van den Hout, "Proust Revisited: Odours as Triggers of Aversive Memories," *Journal of Cognition and Emotion* 26, no. 1(May 2011): 83–92, doi:abs/10.1080/02699931.2011.555475.

7   Fabrice Bartolomei, Stanislas Lagarde, Samuel MédinaVillalon, Aileen Mcgonigal, and Christian G. Bénar, "The "Proust Phenomenon": Odor-Evoked Autobiographical Memories Triggered by Direct Amygdala Stimulation in Human," *Cortex* 90 (2016): 173–75, doi:10.1016/j.cortex .2016.12.005.

8   Athabasca University, "Olfactory Cilia," accessed June 5, 2019, psych.athabascau.ca/html /Psych402/Biotutorials/30/cilia.shtml.

9   Cynthia Deng, "Aromatherapy: Exploring Olfaction," *Yale Scientific*, November 16, 2011, www.yalescientific.org/2011/11/aromatherapy-exploring-olfaction/.

10   Tisserand Institute, "How to Use Essential Oils Safely," accessed June 5, 2019, https://tisserand institute.org/safety/safety-guidelines/.

11   Madeline Vann, "Massage and Emotional Wellness," Everyday Health, last modified December 22, 2009, https://www.everydayhealth.com/emotional-health/the-benefits-of-massage.aspx.

12   Jennifer Peace Rhind, *Aromatherapeutic Blending: Essential Oils in Synergy* (London: Singing Dragon, 2015): 18–19.

13   Liz Fulcher, "Would You Know if You Had an Essential Oil 'Sensitization' Reaction?" Aromatic Wisdom Institute, accessed June 5, 2019, https://aromaticwisdominstitute.com/essential-oil -sensitization/.

14   "Volatile," *Merriam-Webster Dictionary,* accessed June 5, 2019, https://www.merriam-webster .com/dictionary/volatile.

15   Global Market Insights, "Essential Oils Market to Exceed USD 13 Billion by 2024," October 24, 2018, www.globenewswire.com/news-release/2018/10/24/1626070/0/en/Essential-Oils-Market -to-exceed-USD-13-billion-by-2024-Global-Market-Insights-Inc.html.

16   Robert Tisserand and Rodney Young, *Essential Oil Safety: A Guide for Health Care Professionals,* 2nd ed. (Edinburgh: Churchill Livingstone, 2013): 47.

17   Anthea Levi, "Fragrance Sensitivities Can Actually Be Very Severe, Study Finds," *Health,* March 7, 2017, https://www.health.com/allergy/fragrance-sensitivity-health-effects.

18   Abba, "Anointing Oil," accessed June 5, 2019, www.abbaoil.com/t-anointingoilteaching.aspx.

19   Sandhiya Ramaswamy, "The Benefits of Ayurveda Self-Massage 'Abhyanga,'" Chopra Center, accessed June 5, 2019, https://chopra.com/articles/the-benefits-of-ayurveda-self-massage -"abhyanga".

20   Essential Oil Exchange, "Angelica Oil Has Centuries of Historical Use," September 20, 2012, https://blog.essentialoilexchange.com/angelica-oil-has-centuries-of-historical-use/.

21   International Fragrance Association, "Angelica Root," https://ifrafragrance.org/.

22   Eri Watanabe, Kenny Kuchta, Mari Kimura, Hans Wilhelm Rauwald, Tsutomu Kamei, and Jiro Imanishi, "Effects of Bergamot (*Citrus bergamia* [Risso] Wright &Arn.) Essential Oil Aromatherapy on Mood States, Parasympathetic Nervous System Activity, and Salivary Cortisol Levels in 41 Healthy Females," *Complementary Medicine Research* 22, no. 1 (2015): 43–49, doi:10.1159/000380989.

23   International Fragrance Association, "Bergamot Oil Expressed," https://ifrafragrance.org.

24   Patricia Davis, *Subtle Aromatherapy* (Saffron Walden, UK: C. W. Daniel Company, 1996), 51–52.

25   Michele Navarra, Carmen Mannucci, Marisa Delbò, and Gioacchino Calapai, "*Citrus bergamia* Essential Oil: From Basic Research to Clinical Application," *Frontiers in Pharmacology* 6, no. 36 (March 2015), doi:10.3389/fphar.2015.00036.

26   Robert Tisserand, "Citrus Oils and Breast Health," Tisserand Institute, August 10, 2015, https://tisserandinstitute.org/citrus-oils-and-breast-health/.

27   V. M. Linck, A. L. da Silva, M. Figueiró, E. B. Caramão, P. R. H. Moreno, and E. Elisabetsky, "Effects of Inhaled Linalool in Anxiety, Social Interaction and Aggressive Behavior in Mice," *Phytomedicine* 17, no. 8–9 (2010): 679–83, doi:10.1016/j.phymed.2009.10.002.

28   Jennifer Peace Rhind, *Fragrance and Wellbeing: Plant Aromatics and Their Influence on the Psyche* (London: Singing Dragon, 2013), 223.

29   Ming-Chiu Ou, Yu-Fei Lee, Chih-Ching Li, and Shyi-Kuen Wu, "The Effectiveness of Essential Oils for Patients with Neck Pain: A Randomized Controlled Study," *Journal of Alternative and Complementary Medicine* 20, no. 10 (2014): 771–79, doi:10.1089/acm.2013.0453.

30   Malik Hassan Mehmood and Anwarul Hassan Gilani, "Pharmacological Basis for the Medicinal Use of Black Pepper and Piperine in Gastrointestinal Disorders," *Journal of Medicinal Food* 13, no. 5 (2010): 1086–96, doi:10.1089/jmf.2010.1065.

31   Ou et al., "Effectiveness of Essential Oils," 771–79.

32   Jed E. Rose and Frederique M. Behm, "Inhalation of Vapor from Black Pepper Extract Reduces Smoking Withdrawal Symptoms," *Drug and Alcohol Dependence* 34, no. 3 (1994): 225–29, doi:10.1016/0376-8716(94)90160-0.

33   Kurt Schnaubelt, *Medical Aromatherapy: Healing with Essential Oils* (Berkeley, CA: North Atlantic Books, 1999), 187.

34 Peter Holmes, *Aromatica: A Clinical Guide to Essential Oil Therapeutics. Principles and Profiles* (London: Singing Dragon, 2016):149–55.

35 Mahmoud A. Saleh, Shavon Clark, Brooke Woodard, and Suziat Ayomide Deolu-Sobogun, "Antioxidant and Free Radical Scavenging Activities of Essential Oils," *Ethnicity and Disease* 20 (spring 2010): S1-78–S1-82, https://www.ethndis.org/priorsuparchives/ethn-20-01s1-s78.pdf.

36 Whole Spice, "Cardamom: The Queen of Spices," September 30, 2013, https://wholespice.com /blog/cardamom-the-queen-of-spices/.

37 Jade Shutes, "Cardamom: Queen of Spices," New York Institute of Aromatic Studies, August 21, 2018, aromaticstudies.com/cardamom-queen-of-spices/.

38 Tisserand and Young, *Essential Oil Safety,* 232.

39 Singaravel Sengottuvelu, "Cardamom (*Elettariacardamomum Linn. Maton*) Seeds in Health," in *Nuts and Seeds in Health and Disease Prevention,* eds. Victor R. Preedy, Ronald Ross Watson, and Vinood B. Patel (London: Academic Press, 2011), 285–91, doi:10.1016 /b978-0-12-375688-6.10034-9.

40 Peter Holmes, "The Conifer Oils: The Gift of Ancient Times," Snow Lotus, 2005, accessed June 5, 2019, www.snowlotus.org/content/conifer-oils.pdf.

41 *Aromatica*, Holmes, 304–10.

42 Ibid.

43 Stillpoint Aromatics, "Stillpoint's Trauma Remedy Flower Essence (STR)," accessed June 5, 2019, https://www.stillpointaromatics.com/stillpoint-rescue-trauma-remedy-solution?keyword =trauma%20remedy.

44 Bach Centre, "Rock Rose," accessed June 5, 2019, https://www.bachcentre.com/centre/38 /rockrose.htm.

45 Mercedes Verdeguer, M. Amparo Blázquez, and Herminio Boira, "Chemical Composition and Herbicidal Activity of the Essential Oil from a *Cistus ladanifer* L. Population from Spain," *Natural Product Research* 26, no. 17 (2012): 1602–9, doi:10.1080/14786419.2011.592835.

46 Salvatore Battaglia, "Clary Sage," Perfect Potion, 2018, accessed June 5, 2019, www.salvatore battaglia.com.au/wp-content/uploads/2018/08/A4_EssentialOilMonograph_ClarySage _010718.pdf.

47 Holmes, "The Conifer Oils."

48 Scott Gerson, "Aroma Therapy Study," Gerson Institute of Ayurvedic Medicine, accessed May 3, 2019, http://ayurveda.md/research/aroma-therapy-study.

49 Greener Life Club, "Davana Oil," May 24, 2019, http://ayurvedicoils.com/tag/chemical -constituents-of-davana-oil.

50 Garden of Eve, "Elemi Essential Oil, Canarium Luzonicum," accessed June 5, 2019, https://www .gardenofeveskincare.com/gdarticle/elemi-canarium-luzonicum.html.

51 Ibid.

52 Stillpoint Aromatics, "Fragonia TM Essential Oil," accessed June 5, 2019, https://www.stillpoint aromatics.com/fragonia-Agonis-fragrans-0essential-oil-aromatherapy?keyword=fragonia.

53 Salvatore Battaglia, "Fragonia," Perfect Potion, 2018, accessed June 5, 2019, www.perfectpotion .com.au/news/wp-content/uploads/2017/03/A4_EssentialOilOfTheWeek_FRAGONIA.pdf.

54 Shirley Price and Len Price, *Aromatherapy for Health Professionals,* 4th ed. (London: Churchill Livingstone, 2011).

55 Stillpoint Aromatics, "Frankincense Sacra Essential Oil," accessed June 5, 2019, https://www .stillpointaromatics.com/frankincense-sacra-Boswellia-sacra-essential-oil-aromatherapy ?keyword=frankincense.

56 Rhind, *Aromtherapeutic Blending,* 259.

57 Jeanne Rose Aromatherapy Blog, "Galbanum, Resin and More," August 1, 2018, http://jeanne -blog.com/galbanum-resin-more/.

58 Julia Lawless, *The Encyclopedia of Essential Oils: The Complete Guide to the Use of Aromatic Oils in Aromatherapy, Herbalism, Health & Well-Being* (San Francisco: Conari Press, 2013), 255–59.

59 Gabriel Mojay, *Aromatherapy for Healing the Spirit: Restoring Emotional and Mental Balance with Essential Oils* (Rochester, VT: Healing Arts Press, 2000), 133.

60 Katherine A. Hammer and Christine F. Carson, "Antibacterial and Antifungal Activities of Essential Oils," in *Lipids and Essential Oils as Antimicrobial Agents,* ed. Halldor Thormar (West Sussex, UK: 2010), 255–306, doi:10.1002/9780470976623.ch11.

61 Wellness Resources, "D-Limonene: Help for Digestion, Metabolism, Detoxification, Mood," accessed June 6, 2019, https://www.wellnessresources.com/news/d-limonene-help-for-digestion -metabolism-detoxification-anxiety-breast-canc.

62 International Fragrance Association, "Citrus Oils and Other Furocoumarins Containing Essential Oils," June 10, 2015, https://ifrafragrance.org/.

63 Akira Niijima and Katsuya Nagai, "Effect of Olfactory Stimulation with Flavor of Grapefruit Oil and Lemon Oil on the Activity of Sympathetic Branch in the White Adipose Tissue of the Epididymis," *Experimental Biology and Medicine* 228, no. 10 (November 2003): 1190–92, doi:10.1177/153537020322801014.

64 Essential Oil Corsica, "Questions & Answers," Helichrysum Italicum, accessed June 6, 2019, https://helichrysum-italicum.com/q--a-24-w.asp.

65 Davis, *Subtle Aromatherapy.*

66 Franjo Grotenhermen and Ethan B. Russo, eds., *Handbook of Cannabis Therapeutics: From Bench to Bedside* (New York: Routledge, 2006), 191.

67 Vito Mediavilla and Simon Steinemann, "Essential Oil of *Cannabis sativa* L. Strains," International Hemp Association, accessed June 6, 2019, http://www.internationalhempassociation.org/jiha /jiha4208.html.

68 Tapanee Hongratanaworakit, "Stimulating Effect of Aromatherapy Massage with Jasmine Oil," *Natural Product Communications* 5, no. 1 (January 2010): 157–62, doi:10.1177 /1934578x1000500136.

69 International Fragrance Association, "Index of IFRA Standards: Jasmine Absolute," accessed June 5, 2019, https://ifrafragrance.org/.

70 Lawless, *Encyclopedia of Essential Oils,* 25.

71 Donald G. Barceloux, "Camphor (*Cinnamomumcamphora T.* Nees&Eberm.)," in *Medical Toxicology of Natural Substances: Foods, Fungi, Medical Herbs, Plants, and Venomous Animals* (Hoboken, NJ: Wiley, 2008), 407–13.

72 Tisserand and Young, *Essential Oil Safety,* 323.

73   Lawless, *Encyclopedia of Essential Oils*, 118–19.

74   Price and Price, *Aromatherapy for Health Professionals*, 12.

75   Gerhard Buchbauer, Leopold Jirovetz, Walter H. E. Jäger, Helga Dietrich, and Cynthia Plank, "Aromatherapy: Evidence for Sedative Effects of the Essential Oil of Lavender After Inhalation," *Zeitschrift für Naturforschung* 46, no. 11–12 (November 1991): 1067–72.

76   International Fragrance Association, "Citrus Oils." https://ifrafragrance.org.

77   Leslie Moldenauer, "Essential Oils in Water Archives," Lifeholistically, accessed May 3, 2019, http://lifeholistically.com/tag/essential-oils-in-water/.

78   Migiwa Komiya, Takashi Takeuchi, and Etsumori Harada, "Lemon Oil Vapor Causes an Anti-stress Effect via Modulating the 5-HT and DA Activities in Mice," *Behavioural Brain Research* 172, no. 2 (September 2006): 240–49, doi:10.1016/j.bbr.2006.05.006.

79   International Fragrance Association, "Standards Library," accessed April 29, 2019, https://ifrafragrance.org.

80   Yoshinori Kobayashi, Hiroaki Takemoto, ZiqiFua, Emiko Shimizu, and Yukitaka Kinjo, "Enhancement of Pentobarbital-Induced Sleep by the Vaporized Essential Oil of *Citrus keraji* var. *kabuchii* and Its Characteristic Component, γ-Terpinene," *Natural Product Communications* 11, no. 8 (August 2016): 1175–78, doi:10.1177/1934578x1601100836.

81   Mojay, *Healing the Spirit*, 94–95.

82   Fatemeh Bina and Roja Rahimi, "Sweet Marjoram: A Review of Ethnopharmacology, Phytochemistry, and Biological Activities," *Journal of Evidence-Based Complementary & Alternative Medicine* 22, no. 1 (2017): 175–85, doi:10.1177/2156587216650793.

83   Davis, *Subtle Aromatherapy*, 214.

84   Tisserand and Young, *Essential Oil Safety*, 357.

85   Davis, *Subtle Aromatherapy*, 109.

86   Pariya Khodabakhsh, Hamed Shafaroodi, and Jinous Asgarpanah, "Analgesic and Anti-inflammatory Activities of *Citrus aurantium* L. Blossoms Essential Oil (neroli): Involvement of the Nitric Oxide/Cyclic-Guanosine Monophosphate Pathway," *Journal of Natural Medicines* 69, no. 3 (March 2015): 324–31, doi:10.1007/s11418-015-0896-6.

87   Mahdi Jaafarzadeh, Soroor Arman, and Fatemeh Farahbakhsh Pour, "Effect of Aromatherapy with Orange Essential Oil on Salivary Cortisol and Pulse Rate in Children During Dental Treatment: A Randomized Controlled Clinical Trial," *Advanced Biomedical Research* 2, no. 1 (January–March 2013): 1–7, doi:10.4103/2277-9175.107968.

88   Floracopeia, "Ecuador Palo Santo Project," accessed June 5, 2019, https://www.floracopeia.com/ecuador-palo-santo-project.

89   Tisserand and Young, *Essential Oil Safety*, 379.

90   Flor M. Fon-Fay, Jorge A. Pino, Ivones Hernández, Idania Rodeiro, and Miguel D. Fernández, "Chemical Composition and Antioxidant Activity of *Bursera graveolens* (Kunth) Trianaet et Planch Essential Oil from Manabí, Ecuador," *Journal of Essential Oil Research* 31, no. 3 (January 2019): 211–16, doi:10.1080/10412905.2018.1564381.

91   Davis, *Subtle Aromatherapy*.

92 Daniele G. Machado, Manuella P. Kaster, Ricardo W. Binfaré, Munique Dias, Adair R. S. Santos, Moacir G. Pizzolatti, Inês M. C. Brighente, and Ana Lúcia S. Rodrigues, "Antidepressant-like Effect of the Extract from Leaves of *Schinusmolle* L. in Mice: Evidence for the Involvement of the Monoaminergic System," *Progress in Neuro-Psychopharmacology and Biological Psychiatry* 31, no. 2 (March 2007): 421–28, doi:10.1016/j.pnpbp.2006.11.004.

93 Stillpoint Aromatics, "Rhododendron Essential Oil," accessed June 5, 2019, https://www.stillpoint aromatics.com/rhododendron-essential-oil-aromatherapy?keyword=rhododendron.

94 J. D. Roy, A. K. Handique, C. C. Barua, A. Talukdar, F. A. Ahmed, and I. C. Barua, "Evaluation of Phytoconstituents and Assessment of Adaptogenic Activity in Vivo in Various Extracts of *Rhododendron arboreum* (Leaves)," *Indian Journal of Pharmaceutical and Biological Research* 2, no. 2 (April 2014): 49–56, doi:10.30750/ijpbr.2.2.9.

95 Tisserand and Young, *Essential Oil Safety,* 405.

96 New Directions Aromatic Blog, "All about Vetiver Essential Oil," January 31, 2018, https://www .newdirectionsaromatics.com/blog/products/all-about-vetiver-oil.html.

97 Mountain Rose Herbs, "Sandalwood, Australian Essential Oil," accessed June 6, 2019, https://www .mountainroseherbs.com/products/sandalwood-australian-essential-oil/profile.

98 Mojay, *Healing the Spirit,* 116–17.

99 Holmes, "The Conifer Oils."

100 Mojay, *Healing the Spirit,* 118–19.

101 Holmes, *Aromatica,* 353–61.

102 Irinéia Baretta, Regiane Américo Felizardo, Vanessa Fávero Bimbato, Maísa Gonçalves Jorge dos Santos, Candida Aparecida Leite Kassuya, Arquimedes Gasparotto Jr., Cássia Reginada Silva, Sara Marchesande Oliveira, Juliano Ferreira, and Roberto Andreatini, "Anxiolytic-like Effects of Acute and Chronic Treatment with *Achillea millefolium* L. Extract," *Journal of Ethno-pharmacology* 40, no. 1 (March 2012): 46–54, https://www.sciencedirect.com/science/article /pii/S0378874111008567.

103 Holmes, *Aromatica,* 364.

104 Tisserand and Young, *Essential Oil Safety,* 477.

105 Mojay, *Healing the Spirit,* 133.

106 In-Hee Kim, Chan Kim, Kayeon Seong, Myung-Haeng Hur, Heon Man Lim, and Myeong Soo Lee, "Essential Oil Inhalation on Blood Pressure and Salivary Cortisol Levels in Prehypertensive and Hypertensive Subjects," *Evidence-Based Complementary and Alternative Medicine* 2012 (2012): 1–9, doi:10.1155/2012/984203.

107 Schnaubelt, *Medical Aromatherapy,* 187.

108 Seyedemaryam Lotfipur-Rafsanjani, Ali Ravari, Zohreh Ghorashi, Saiedeh Haji-Maghsoudi, Jafar Akbarinasab, and Reza Bekhradi, "Effects of Geranium Aromatherapy Massage on Premenstrual Syndrome: A Clinical Trial," *International Journal of Preventive Medicine* 9, no. 1 (2018): 98, doi:10.4103/ijpvm.ijpvm_40_16.

109 Rhind, *Aromatherapeutic Blending,* 259.

110 Niijima and Nagai, "Olfactory Stimulation," 1190–92.

111 Rafie Hamidpour, Soheila Hamidpour, Mohsen Hamidpour, and Mina Shahlari. "Frankincense (乳香 Rǔ Xiāng; Boswellia Species): From the Selection of Traditional Applications to the Novel Phytotherapy for the Prevention and Treatment of Serious Diseases," *Journal of Traditional and Complementary Medicine* 3, no. 4 (October–December 2013): 221–26, doi:10.4103/2225-4110.119723.

112 Bahar Gholipour, "A Parent's Touch Actually Transforms A Baby's Brain," Huffington Post, July 29, 2016, https://www.huffpost.com/entry/parents-touch-child-brain_n_579ae4c0e4b08a8e8b5d83cd.

113 "One Percent of Americans Visit Doctors Each Year to Manage Health Problems Caused by Medication," PsycEXTRA Dataset, 2005, doi:10.1037/e556202006-020.

114 Stillpoint Aromatics, "Emotional Well Being Kit," accessed June 6, 2019, https://www.stillpointaromatics.com/emotional-well-being-kit-fragonia-rhododendron-white-ginger-lily-bergamot-essential-oils.

115 Mayo Clinic, "Seasonal Affective Disorder (SAD)," October 25, 2017, https://www.mayoclinic.org/diseases-conditions/seasonal-affective-disorder/symptoms-causes/syc-20364651.

116 Teruhisa Komori, Ryoichi Fujiwara, Masahiro Tanida, Junichi Nomura, and Mitchel M. Yokoyama, "Effects of Citrus Fragrance on Immune Function and Depressive States," *Neuroimmunomodulation* 2, no. 3 (May 1995): 174–80, doi:10.1159/000096889.

117 Shan Dong and Tim J. C. Jacob, "Combined Non-adaptive Light and Smell Stimuli Lowered Blood Pressure, Reduced Heart Rate and Reduced Negative Affect," *Physiology & Behavior* 156 (2016): 94–105, doi:10.1016/j.physbeh.2016.01.013.

118 Janmejai K. Srivastava, Eswar Shankar, and Sanjay Gupta, "Chamomile: A Herbal Medicine of the Past with a Bright Future (Review)," *Molecular Medicine Reports* 3, no. 6 (2010): 895–901, doi:10.3892/mmr.2010.377.

119 Tisserand, "Citrus Oils and Breast Health."

120 Michelle Fondin, "The Root Chakra: Muladhara," Chopra Center, accessed June 5, 2019, chopra.com/articles/the-root-chakra-muladhara.

121 Michelle Fondin, "Awaken Your Creativity Chakra: Svadhisthana," Chopra Center, accessed June 5, 2019, chopra.com/articles/awaken-your-creativity-chakra-svadhisthana.

122 Michelle Fondin, "Find Power and Warrior Energy in Your Third Chakra," Chopra Center, January 15, 2015, chopra.com/articles/find-power-and-warrior-energy-in-your-third-chakra.

123 Michelle Fondin, "Open Yourself to Love with the Fourth Chakra," Chopra Center, accessed June 5, 2019, chopra.com/articles/open-yourself-to-love-with-the-fourth-chakra.

124 Michelle Fondin, "Speak Your Inner Truth with the Fifth Chakra," Chopra Center, accessed June 5, 2019, chopra.com/articles/speak-your-inner-truth-with-the-fifth-chakra.

125 Michelle Fondin, "Trust Your Intuition with the Sixth Chakra," Chopra Center, May 26, 2015, chopra.com/articles/trust-your-intuition-with-the-sixth-chakra.

126 Michelle Fondin, "Connect to the Divine with the Seventh Chakra," Chopra Center, accessed June 5, 2019, chopra.com/articles/connect-to-the-divine-with-the-seventh-chakra.

Acknowledgments

First, I'd like to thank my mom, stepdad, and sister for always believing in me, even when I struggled to believe in myself. You are my inspirations and have shown me that anything is possible. Words can never express how much I love you.

A massive thanks to my dear friends who have helped me through every step of this journey: Ashley Glassman, Sam Brown, Heather Morris, Brook Reed, Dina VanDecker-Tibbs, Jennifer Jeffries, Haly JensenHof, Elizabeth Russell, and so many others. True friends are worth their weight in gold. I'm glad I found you all and am so grateful for our friendships.

To every single person who has helped me along my journey in life and my career, including those at Callisto Media who made this dream a beautiful reality: Even if I have not been able to name you all here, know that your support and the life lessons you taught me mean everything to me.

Thank you to my boys, Aiden and Owen, who have endured endless takeout meals, altered schedules, and more chores than they care to count. I especially want to thank Aiden, who has grown up so quickly and spent hours helping me do research and acting as my sounding board. He has been integral to bringing this labor of love to fruition. Aiden and Owen, I love you both to the moon and back.

Last, but definitely not least, thanks to you, my awesome reader, for coming on this journey of emotional healing. This is but one of many steps on your way to wellness.

About the Author

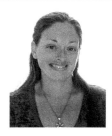 **LESLIE MOLDENAUER** is the owner of Lifeholistically LLC, a trusted online educational resource that covers essential oil safety and encompasses all that natural living has to offer. She is an experienced aromatherapist with a practice firmly rooted in research and science who has been working with essential oils for more than a decade. Leslie earned her Associate of Applied Science degree in Complementary Alternative Medicine with Aromatherapy Specialization from the American College of Healthcare Sciences. She also has received extensive training as a Certified Aromatherapy Practitioner and Certified Holistic Nutritional Consultant in addition to her work with plant medicine, energy medicine, meditation, yoga, and stress management.

CPSIA information can be obtained
at www.ICGtesting.com
Printed in the USA
BVHW051936060919
557465BV00001B/1/P

9 781641 525466